THE HEALTHY LUNCHBOX

FIONA BECKETT

THE HEALTHY LUNCHBOX
FIONA BECKETT

GRUB STREET · LONDON

Dedication

To my children William, Jo, Kate and Flyn who, I have to confess, didn't always get lunchboxes as exciting as these . . .

Acknowledgements

Thanks first and foremost to Anne Dolamore of Grub Street, whose brilliant idea this book was and who pushed the project through with her customary energy and drive. Photographer Michelle Garrett who made the lunchboxes look so great and Lizzie Ballantyne for her lively, creative design for the book. Ros Ellis for spreading the word about it, Kerry Torrens for keeping me on the nutritional straight and narrow, Helen Barker-Benfield for checking the recipes and to my niece Anna Pierssené, a primary school teacher, for feedback from the sharp end. And to the many parents I spoke to about the project especially Donna and Tracy.

Published in 2005 by
Grub Street
4 Rainham Close
London
SW11 6SS
Email: food@grubstreet.co.uk
Web: www.grubstreet.co.uk

Text copyright © Fiona Beckett
Copyright this edition © Grub Street 2005
Photography by Michelle Garrett
Book design by Lizzie Ballantyne
Jacket design by Hugh Adams
Food styling and preparation by Fiona Beckett
Nutritional analysis of recipes by Kerry Torrens

British Library Cataloguing in Publication Data
Beckett, Fiona
The healthy lunchbox
1. Lunchbox cookery 2. Children - nutrition 3. School children
- Food
I. Title
641.5'34

ISBN-10: 1 904943 23 3

Printed and bound in Spain by Bookprint, S.L., Barcelona

CONTENTS

FOREWORD

If your child takes a packed lunch to school every day, by the time they leave at 16 you will have prepared well over two thousand lunchboxes. Considerably more if you have several children. Combine that with the pressure of seeing them off every morning and getting yourself out to work and you can see why so many parents take the line of least resistance and send their kids off with packets of crisps and chocolate bars in their boxes.

Lunch however is a critical meal on which your child depends for a third of their daily nutritional requirements so it's not an exaggeration to say that how well your child does at school depends on what you provide for them in their lunchbox. If you wouldn't dream of eating yourself what your child takes to school you're almost certainly giving them the wrong things...

I'm not underestimating the difficulties of introducing changes particularly if you have children with allergies and intolerances or rigid ideas about what they like and dislike. But what I've tried to do in this book is to offer some new and inspiring ideas in the form of 10 different types of lunchbox. As you'll see from the way the lunchboxes are organised they're based - with one or two exceptions - on themed approaches to food rather than strict age groups. After all some 5 year olds are much more open to new foods than some 15 year olds.

You'll find the low-down on the lunchboxes on pages 18-36 and the recipes for the suggested meals are on the pages following. They are all cross referenced so for example you can see that 'hummus' listed in a number of the lunchboxes is marked with * to show there is a recipe for it in the book.

The contents of the lunchboxes I have created shouldn't in any way be regarded as rigid. A teenage girl may fancy the little fruit jellies in My First Lunchbox or the 'fishy hummus' in The Big Dipper. A teenage boy won't say no to the Chewy Banana Flapjacks in the Green Lunchbox. Children who eat wheat may well enjoy the Jewelled Rice Salad in the 'Free From' section and an adventurous 7 year old will probably love the Cajun burgers in the Hero Lunchbox. I hope his parents will too.

I'm not of course suggesting you should spend every evening whipping up culinary masterpieces but if you take a holistic view of the family's diet - seeing evening meals as an opportunity to create leftovers for the next day - you'll find it's surprisingly easy to make improvements not only in your children's but in your own lunchtime eating habits too. You will, of course, make life immeasurably easier for yourself if all the family members eat the same meals (see Lunchbox Psychology p. 11). The idea that children need separate and different food choices is a brilliant strategy on the part of food manufacturers to increase the amount you spend on the family shopping basket each week.

Good shopping, in fact, is what good eating depends upon. Even if you make none of the recipes in this book but if you choose the products you buy more carefully and incorporate a greater amount of fresh fruit and vegetables into your child's diet, you'll be doing them a huge favour.

Finally, the good news is that in the current climate you stand a much better chance of making a healthy lunchbox acceptable to your child than you would a couple of years ago; there is a huge amount of choice and many supermarkets stock healthy and organic ranges now as a matter of course. Also you have the support of both government and schools in your crusade as they, at long last, are determined to see children eat more healthily.

Fiona Beckett

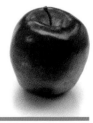

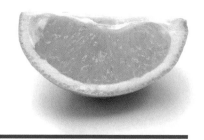

A BALANCED LUNCH

WHY SO MANY LUNCHBOXES ARE UNHEALTHY

A recent survey by the Food Standards Agency showed that 9 out of 10 children took packed lunches to school that were too high in saturated fat, sugar and salt. It doesn't surprise me. You only have to look at the sections of the supermarket shelves that are devoted to food that is targeted at kids, particularly snacks, confectionery and dairy products, to see why.

The shocking truth is that the majority of the products promoted for lunchboxes couldn't be less suitable. Fruit-flavoured dairy products that contain little or no fruit and far too much sugar. Bars that are far too sweet and simply give a short-term sugar rush. Cold meats and cheese products that contain scant amounts of lean meat or cheese and far too much salt and chemical additives. Drinks that amount to little more than sugared water.

Worst of all are the ready-made lunchboxes with lengthy shelf lives. The companies who make them cynically give the impression by listing the vitamins and minerals they've added that they're balanced and healthy but with their total absence of fresh ingredients they're anything but. It's almost got to the stage where if the product has a silly name and cartoon character on the pack you'd be well advised to steer clear of it.

Even products that appear more wholesome are in many cases less than ideal. Apparently healthy cereal bars are often lamentably low in fruit or fibre. Some fruit juices needlessly contain added sugar. 'Low fat' crisps that are still way too high in saturated fat. No wonder the average parent is confused.

WHAT DO CHILDREN ACTUALLY NEED?

Lunch is a vital pit-stop during the school day, an opportunity to restore flagging energy and boost concentration. Children who don't eat a proper meal struggle to take in information in the second half of the day and may suffer from behavioural problems. Their overall health can also suffer if they regularly do without key vitamins and minerals like calcium and iron. A lack of iron, for example, can easily make teenage girls anaemic, listless and depressed.

Lunch should not only constitute a third of a child's daily calorie intake (the officially recommended amount is 30%) but roughly a third of a child's daily intake of each of the food groups they need for a balanced diet. The Caroline Walker Trust nutritional guidelines for school meals which are the ones school caterers officially work to – indicate that carbohydrate should be the backbone of the meal (50%) and that it should contain no more than 11% saturated fat or sugar. It should provide 30% of the child's protein requirements and between 30-40% of the iron, calcium, vitamin A and vitamin C they need for the day.

How much of each food each child needs depends on their age, size and level of activity. There's obviously a huge difference between a 4 year old girl and a 16 year old boy as the chart below shows.

Age Group	Average Height (cm)		Average Weight (kg)		Calories Needed		Protein (g)	
4-6 years	110		17.5		1715 -1545		19.7	
7-10 years	127		25.5		1970-1740		28.3	
11-14 years	148		43.4		2220-1845		41.65	
15-18 years	Male 170	Female 161	Male 64.5	Female 55.5	Male 2755	Female 2110	Male 55.2	Female 45.0

WHAT A HEALTHY PACKED LUNCH SHOULD INCLUDE

I don't for a moment want to get away from the idea that food should be enjoyable but if you take the view that everything in your child's lunchbox needs to earn its place or in other words that nothing should be included that's of zero nutritional value you won't go far wrong.

Carbohydrate
Kids need carbs to give them energy. The most usual source is a sandwich which 82% of children take to school according to the Food Standards Agency's latest lunchbox survey (see p. 61) but they can equally well be provided by pasta, rice, noodles or couscous and by beans, chickpeas and other pulses (see below). Wholewheat bread and other grains, which count as complex carbohydrates are better sources of fibre than white bread and will boost your child's energy longer. Wholewheat pitta breads are an excellent and inexpensive choice. (For wheat-free diets see p. 28)

Protein
This is vital for healthy growth. The principal sources are meat, fish, dairy products and eggs and, for vegetarians, tofu, nuts and pulses such as beans and chickpeas. Bread also contains a useful amount. As meals shouldn't consist of more than 11% saturated fat your emphasis should be on lean meat such as ham and chicken rather than manufactured meat products such as chicken roll or salami. Children's need for protein varies with their age and size but may be less than you think. A 4-6 year old needs just fewer than 20g or 6.5g at lunchtime, a requirement easily met by a small wholemeal roll filled with 25g of chicken or cheese. Oily fish such as salmon and sardines are not only a good source of protein but contain omega 3 oils which improve mood and academic performance.

A low fat **DAIRY** product such as cheese, fromage frais, yoghurt or a milk or yoghurt drink like a smoothie may constitute the protein component of the meal or be there to boost its calcium content, again crucial for growth and calm behaviour. Watch out though for the sugar content of many commercial yoghurt and fromage frais products that are targeted at children. (For dairy-free alternatives see the 'Free From' lunchbox on p. 28)

2 portions of Fruit and/or Vegetables
If your child is to eat at least 5 portions of fruit and vegetables a day then 2 of them need to be consumed at lunchtime or in breaks. One could be a fruit juice though it's preferable if fruit is fresh, seasonal and either organic or locally grown otherwise its vitamin content may be diminished. There's no reason though why it can't be incorporated in a smoothie or a home-made jelly (see p. 58)

It's easy enough to slip salad vegetables such as tomatoes, lettuce and cucumber into a sandwich or to cut up some carrot sticks and peppers to go with a dip (see the Big Dipper Lunchbox on p. 20). It's important to include as many different fruit and vegetables as you can get away with so your child gets a full range of different nutrients (see Lunchbox Psychology p. 11).

Water
The biggest favour you can do your child is to give them a taste for plain water, which is essential to keep them hydrated and sustain their concentration. The school will no doubt provide it but if the taste of the local tap water is unpalatable you might want to send them to

school with a small bottle of mineral water. Any other drink such as fruit juice or milk should be additional to that.

A between-meals snack

For morning breaks or immediately after school. Not crisps please which have little nutritional value. Dried fruits such as raisins or apricots, nuts or seed mixes or a healthy bar based on oats or dried fruits are ideal. Or a piece of fresh fruit. Older children may need something more substantial especially after sustained physical activity – an extra sandwich or roll or a couple of oatcakes and cheese. And there's no harm in an occasional treat like a home-baked muffin or a piece of tiffin (see p. 59) or even a small bar or square or two of plain dark chocolate (provided your child's school allows it).

LUNCHBOX BADDIES AND HOW TO AVOID THEM

Ironically many of the products that are most heavily marketed to children contain excessive amounts of ingredients that are bad for them – salt, sugar and saturated fat. If you buy them in addition to everyday products that also contain significant levels of these ingredients your child will end up having far more than they need.

Salt

Recommended limits for salt are 6g for children over 11 years, 5g for 7-10 year olds and just 3g for 4-6 year olds. It's easy to accumulate these lower levels in lunch alone if you don't watch out. Ham and cheese, for example contain significant amounts of salt. So, more surprisingly, does bread – which can contain up to 2g per 100g (levels over 1.25g per 100g are considered high and as an average slice of bread weighs about 50g per slice, two slices making up a sandwich may contribute around 2g of salt). Often salt is expressed as sodium on nutritional labels which can be confusing. You have to multiply by 2.5 to get the salt content. Avoid adding salt, which can routinely store up long term health problems. You'll find your child's (and your own) taste for it diminishes and that another ingredient such as lemon juice or onion will do the job instead (see www.salt.gov.uk).

Sugar

Another ingredient that food manufacturers sneak into products where you least expect it, such as sandwich fillings as well as children's yoghurts and drinks. See where it appears on the ingredients list and be aware that it's not always labelled as such.

It can be listed as sucrose, glucose, dextrose or corn syrup. More than 10g of sugars per 100g of product is considered high. Excessive sugar is best avoided because it contributes to tooth decay and can result in mood and concentration swings. Again, only add it as needed, to sweeten slightly unripe fruit for example.

Saturated fat

Fat is not all bad and that's especially true for children who need the energy fats provide and vitamins they disperse round the body. The types to limit are saturated animal-derived fats like whole milk, cream, butter and red meat which should make up no more than 10% of your child's calorie intake and so-called 'trans-fats', artificially created fats that occur in products such as commercial biscuits and cakes. On the other hand unsaturated fats such as olive oil, the fats you find in nuts and seeds and in oily fish are all hugely beneficial. The message? Stick to lean meat and low fat dairy foods (though younger children should not have skimmed milk), use spreads like butter sparingly and include plenty of nuts and seeds among your snacks.

Additives

Some children are more sensitive to additives than others but they've certainly been linked convincingly with behavioural problems, so I would avoid as a general principle products that contain artificial colours and flavourings (especially MSG) or which contain long lists of E numbers – which alarmingly includes a significant number of products that are marketed to children. Organic ingredients and ready-made foods are generally much better in this respect but still not as good as food you make from scratch yourself.

READING THE LABEL

It's always worth checking the labels of the foods you buy – difficult though that can be. They are sometimes printed so small that it's impossible to read them without a magnifying glass which can make you look slightly demented as you go round the supermarket. Sharp-eyed children may be able to help you – which has the added bonus that they too become more conscious of what's in the food they eat. Ingredients are listed with the ones that take up the greatest proportion of the total first. Look out particularly for the actual amount of a healthy ingredient that's pictured on the label. The fruit content, for example, can be almost negligible.

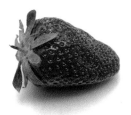

LUNCHBOX PSYCHOLOGY

Children are all different but by and large what they want from their lunchbox (fast food that can be wolfed in 5 minutes) is never going to be what their parents – and teachers – want for them: food that is healthy, sustaining and brain-boosting. Kids are fiendishly good at throwing up a whole raft of obstructive devices, to prevent you realising your aim, from arbitrary objections to dislike of specific ingredients to emotional blackmail (Sally's mum lets her have crisps in her lunchbox . . .) Here are some strategies that may help you cope:

12 DEVIOUS WAYS
TO A HEALTHIER LUNCHBOX

1 **LIMIT CHOICE** Never ask the open-ended question what would you like in your lunchbox? Children find it difficult to envisage foods they haven't tried and will almost certainly come up with something they've had several hundred times before. A better tactic is to offer a choice between two or three options or get your child to help you plan a whole week's lunches.

2 **INVOLVE** your child as much as possible in preparing their lunchbox. Even from an early age kids can help in the kitchen – helping to put the topping on a pizza or mixing together ingredients for flapjacks. Older children can be entrusted with chopping vegetables for salads and salsas or whizzing up smoothies and spreads. Give them as much responsibility as they'll take, encouraging older children to help younger ones. Sunday afternoons are a good time to get preparation done for the week.

If this sounds impossibly idyllic, especially with sullen teenagers don't despair. Not all kids (or parents, come to that) are budding Jamie Olivers. With some kids the request may be better pitched as an invitation to keep you company in the kitchen while you're preparing the lunchbox(es) and just ask them to do the odd job, such as finding you an ingredient you need while they're there. If they associate the preparation of food with an opportunity to get you on their own for a chat they're more likely to have a positive attitude to family meals as a whole, not just lunchboxes

3 **BE SENSITIVE** while sticking to your guns about sending your child to school with healthy food though be aware that there are things they may find embarrassing. Even a child who happily eats food flavoured with garlic at home will not necessarily welcome it – or other smelly ingredients like raw onion, strong cheese or fish – in their lunchbox. Some children are more self-conscious than others about leftovers. Gnawing on a cold chicken leg may make them stand out from the crowd whereas cutting the meat off and tucking it in a sandwich or pitta bread would not.

If your child's lunchbox comes back with half the contents uneaten try and find out what the problem is. Has another child made a disparaging remark about it? Was it genuinely something they disliked and was that the taste or the texture? It may just be a question of presentation. Too many dinky little containers may make your child an object of fun. If you gave them an all-in-one dish such as a salad it might not be remarked upon. Give some thought to what you call dishes too. If you think your child might be sent up for taking chicken fajitas to school just call them chicken wraps.

Some parents like to drop a message into their child's lunchbox but beware sloppy messages, however well meant, can also make your child cringe. Try and make them funny rather than sentimental or send them from the family pet. Small children like awful puns and bad cracker-style jokes. Encourage them to bring one back for you in their empty lunchbox. Older children may appreciate a philosophical quote or a line of poetry on a particularly tough day so that they know you're thinking of them – but again, do it discreetly.

4 **GIVE GROUND** on the container itself. So long as it's practical, robust and hygienic it doesn't matter what sort of 'box', bag or other container your child takes to school. However tacky you may think it is allow them to choose their own.

5 **SHARE YOUR CONCERNS** about junk foods. Don't just arbitrarily ban certain products, explain why. Even small children can understand that it's better not to eat things that result in them having to go to the dentist more often or that living off crisps doesn't fill them up. Point out how little (if any) real fruit there is in the heavily advertised yoghurt they want to buy. Point out articles to teenagers about how poor diet causes skin problems. Show kids positive images of healthy looking sportsmen and women who eat lots of fresh fruit and vegetables. Watch 'fat camp' type programmes about overweight children together and discuss the problems it causes for them. Don't be obsessive about it, obviously, but take the opportunity to have a dialogue with your kids about healthy eating whenever the opportunity naturally occurs.

6 **DON'T REWARD** children with unhealthy foods. It's easy to fall into the trap of offering an unhealthy snack as a reward for eating an unpopular food or trying something new. But the message that gives out is that these are special foods. It's much better to make a treat a home baked cake or biscuit or a luxury, like a sandwich made with prawns or smoked salmon. Or to make the reward entirely unrelated to food. An agreement to try five new foods might be rewarded by a family trip to the cinema, for example. Or a book or magazine your child particularly wants. Some kind of incentive is likely to be needed particularly at the beginning when you start making substantial changes to the lunchbox.

7 **BE CONSISTENT**, don't give up in exasperation and agree to foods like chocolate bars and crisps that you've previously outlawed. Don't have food lying around at home that you wouldn't be happy to see in your child's lunchbox. And make sure that everyone who might be involved in preparing your child's lunchbox – your partner, your parents, your in-laws, your ex and his/her partner – adhere to the same rules

8 **TEAM UP** with other parents. Your child will find it easier to eat healthily if his or her friends do too. You will almost certainly find that his friends' parents are keen to improve their child's diet. At the very least you could probably all benefit from swapping tips and strategies so that none of them, for example, takes in crisps or confectionery. If you're exceptionally well organised you could even devise a rota system where one parent in the school run makes all the lunchboxes for a week then gets a couple of weeks off. Or one parent – or older child – who enjoys preparing food does it regularly and gets paid for it.

9 **ENCOURAGE** your child to be more adventurous about food by going out as a family to eat in different types of restaurants, especially ethnic ones such as Greek, Indian or Chinese. If you're out shopping together at the weekend stop for a sandwich or a snack somewhere you know there will be unusual salads, breads and sandwich fillings. Shop, where you can, in markets or smaller shops where you can taste before you buy. If you buy something really delicious like strawberries or raspberries, for a dinner party or another meal with friends, save some for the kids.

10 **EAT THE SAME FOOD** as your children as far as possible. By sharing family meals you stand a better chance of extending your children's repertoire of foods, discouraging faddiness and encouraging them to eat the same things. It also helps to try unfamiliar foods first at home rather than road-testing them in the lunchbox.

11 **DON'T EXPECT** miracles overnight. Bad habits take time to break. Having outlawed the foods you object to most strongly (crisps, confectionery and fizzy drinks) take a more gradual approach to replacing other foods with healthier alternatives. White bread for

example can be replaced by fortified white bread with grains as a stepping stone to wholemeal. Substitute choc chip bars for chocolate ones on the way to bars that are full of sustaining nuts, seeds and dried fruits. Dilute fruit juice progressively with water until you manage to persuade your child that water tastes better. Gradually reduce the amounts of salt and sugar you add to favourite foods (good for all the family not just kids).

12 KEEP TRYING foods that have been rejected, in another guise if necessary. Kids who don't like raw peppers for example may enjoy them roasted and vice versa. Fruits that are blitzed in a smoothie may be accepted when they wouldn't be in their raw form. Develop the art of concealing unloved ingredients in dishes your child will like (see Just-Like-Tuna Pâté on p. 42 and the Tomato (and four other vegetables) Soup on p. 38).

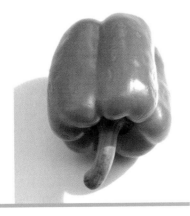

OVERWEIGHT, UNDERWEIGHT AND SUPER-FUSSY CHILDREN

It's particularly hard to cater for kids who have an unhealthy relationship with food – either because they're over or underweight or because they're exceptionally fussy. Extreme examples of all conditions need professional help but there are things you can do to coax or cajole your child out of bad habits.

With overweight children it's often a question of weaning them off fatty and sugary foods, not easy, admittedly, as they're likely to be particularly self-conscious about being seen to eat anything that might draw attention to their size. Try the 'I don't want to be different lunchbox' on p. 22, make sure that the contents of the box are sustaining and look substantial. Give them mayo-free sandwiches crammed with plenty of veg and home baked flapjacks as a filling treat. Make sure to send them off with a good breakfast and promise a (healthy) treat when they get home. And – common sense, of course – encourage them to take more exercise.

Underweight children who eat less than they need – a condition prevalent among teenage girls- is often an issue of control so try and give your kids as much responsibility as you can for preparing their own food and share the plentiful information that is available about the foods they need to remain healthy. You can almost certainly find some chink in their armour – such as a sweet tooth which can be satisfied by a real fruit muffin – on which you can build a more sustaining diet. (See the Lite Lunchbox on p. 34)

Picky eating, by contrast, is generally a phenomenon of younger childhood, and one they normally grow out of if it's not habitually indulged. It helps to make food look as attractive as possible. A lunchbox that looks the same day after day does little to encourage adventurousness. Deals can also be struck. The much loved jam sandwich can be included once or twice a week so long as your child agrees to give a couple of other foods a go. Try a different approach like the Big Dipper Lunchbox on p. 20 or Italian lunchbox on p. 24.

Above all make sure your own behaviour – whether it's an excessive concern about weight or a tendency to tuck into unhealthy snacks yourself – isn't creating a negative model for your child's attitude to food.

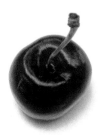

PRACTICAL HINTS AND TIPS

CAN'T COOK/WON'T COOK – TIPS FOR THE HARD-PRESSED WORKING PARENT

If you don't want to cook these days, you don't need to. The whole food industry is dedicated to providing food we can put straight on to our plates – or in our lunchboxes. You can buy in every single component your child needs – sandwiches, salads, little bags of dipping vegetables, dinky fruit salads – at a price.

If you're willing to rustle up a few sandwiches, that too is easy. Every kind of meat you can imagine comes sliced; cheese comes grated, salad leaves ready washed in bags. It's not a problem.

The only real issue is how healthy it is. Many ready-made foods – even ones that appear to be healthy – come with elevated levels of fat, salt and sugar that may make your apparently healthy choice an unhealthy one. And many products that are specifically marketed for children's lunchboxes are shockingly bad.

You do need, if you're concerned about what your child eats, to wise up on what constitutes excessive levels of fat, sugar and salt. (see page 20). The amount of premium ingredients such as meat or chicken may also be quite meagre and of dubious provenance. There aren't many organic sandwiches, sandwich spreads or salads around,

for example. The chicken or egg that is used is not going to be free range unless it says so on the packaging. So if you don't like to cook at least shop well. Products I like are listed opposite.

The other concern is making sure your child has a sufficiently varied diet. Pre-prepared food has a similarity in taste (usually highly seasoned) and texture (more often than not soft) that may stunt your child's palate and make them more resistant to trying a variety of foods.

Even if you haven't time to prepare it yourself it's worth seeing if you can incorporate some kind of home-prepared food in your child's lunchbox. Is there someone you know who enjoys cooking and who you could pay (either in money or in kind) to do the job for you? No need to feel guilty about that – many people offload their housework and their ironing so why not if you can afford it? It could provide some useful additional income for a pensioner or a parent at home with young children. Or maybe you can do it on the basis of barter if you have some skill you can offer them. Either way it's likely to be a more economical proposition if you can persuade all your children to eat the same thing on any one day.

HEALTHIER BOUGHT-IN OPTIONS

Sandwiches
Sandwiches made with wholemeal bread will provide more sustained energy than ones made with white bread. In general it's better to choose ones without mayo unless you're buying premium quality sandwiches – it can constitute a surprising amount of the filling. That applies to sandwich spreads too. Always choose a sandwich that has a decent amount of veg in it (not just sweetcorn). Don't choose sandwiches with fillings that are high in salt (e.g. ham and cheese) more than a couple of times a week.

Salads
Again better without mayo. Check out the salt and sugar levels too.

Yoghurts, fromage frais and other dairy products
Most products that are targeted at children have far too high levels of sugar and not nearly as much fruit as the product label suggests. One probiotic yoghurt drink I looked at, targeted at small children, contained only 1% fruit puree. Organic dairy products are generally much better in this respect. The Little Rachel's Organic range (which has 22% fruit content) is a good example.

Bars + Biscuits
Often look much healthier than they are, especially the branded cereal bars which, despite being reinforced with vitamins and minerals are generally high in sugar and saturated fat. Look for ones that are based on sustaining oats, nuts (if your child can tolerate them) and dried fruits such as Geo bars, Eat Natural and Fruitus. (Healthier options tend to be sold in the special diets section of supermarkets but check the label.) Fruit-based school bars and flakes such as Fruitbowl and Jordan's Frusli, while useful for vegans and children who are dairy- and wheat-intolerant, shouldn't be regarded as a substitute for fresh fruit.

Snacks
There is no such thing as a healthy crisp. Reduced fat still means a lot of fat. Even root vegetable crisps contain a significant amount. Surprisingly Twiglets are not a bad option though higher in salt than they should ideally be and unsalted, unflavoured tortilla chips are pretty healthy, especially if dunked in a fresh tomato salsa. (You can make your own tortilla chips by cutting up soft tortillas and baking in the oven till crisp.) Try and get your child used to unsalted nuts, dried fruits (Oxfam does a particularly good range) and seed mixes like Munchy.

Drinks
It may be a natural instinct to put a carton of juice in your child's lunchbox but make sure it is pure, unsweetened juice not a 'juice drink.' And don't include more than one as they're naturally high in sugar. Many fruit drinks targeted at children boast no added sugar or artificial colours but in my view amount to little more than flavoured, chemically sweetened water. Make sure you include a bottle of water too.

Don't on any account fall for the all-in-one lunchboxes that are targeted at young children which are shockingly poor quality and far too high in salt.

BUDGET LUNCHBOXES

How to create a healthy lunchbox on the cheap
Having written two cookery books for students I've learnt a good deal about shopping on a tight budget. And the most important lesson is how much you can save if everyone eats the same thing. £1 for example won't go far if you allow each child the luxury of having his or her favourite sandwich fillings every day. But £4 for four identical (or more or less identical) lunchboxes buys a great deal.

Other money-saving tips
> Avoid pre-prepared products such as bags of salad leaves and ready-sliced or grated cheese. A fresh lettuce doesn't take a moment to wash and is about a quarter the price of a bag.
> Buy a cool looking branded water bottle then, once your child has drunk the contents, keep filling it up with tap water.
> Buy fresh produce loose rather than pre-packed. You'll be amazed at the difference if you check out the unit cost (the cost per 100g or per kilo) and you only need buy as much as you need.
> Buy ingredients in season. Citrus fruits for example are much more expensive in summer, salad veg like cucumber and spring onions ridiculously pricey in winter.
> Incorporate some sustaining pulse-based salads into the weekly menu. A chickpea or mixed bean salad for instance can be cheaper than a sandwich and is highly nutritious.
> Resist pressure to buy heavily advertised brands. You pay for those ads.
> Be aware of the premium you pay for fashionable ingredients. Cheeses like feta, goats' cheese and mozzarella, for example, are far more expensive than British regional cheeses or less well known products like Quark (an excellent German low fat cheese).

Wraps are much pricier than pitta bread.

> Buy ingredients like nuts and dried fruits in the largest quantities you can afford and divide them up yourself into portions – much cheaper than buying individual child-sized packets.
> Shop towards the end of the day when shops are clearing out foods that have reached or are about to reach their sell-by date. (Use them up quickly, obviously.)
> Plan ahead (see below). You can make ingredients go further if you use them more than once – for example a packet of ham could go to make sandwiches one day, a pasta salad the next and a frittata the following day.

PLANNING AHEAD

Even if you don't stick to it rigidly it helps to have some kind of a plan of what you're going to eat for the week – or for the next few days at least. For a number of good reasons:

> You stand a much better chance of giving your family a varied and balanced diet.
> You don't have to go to the shops so often.
> It helps you economise and avoid wastage.
> You give yourself a negotiating tool. A child who is disappointed at the content of their lunchbox or supper one day may be happier by seeing their favourite meal is coming up in a couple of days' time.

Many meals can easily be turned into lunchbox ingredients for the next day.

> Leftover pasta and rice can be turned into a healthy salad (see p. 45 and 48).
> Cooked chicken and other meats can be incorporated into salads or used to fill sandwiches and wraps (p 54).
> Cold sausages (with high meat content) make a great additional snack for hungry teenage boys.
> Cold roast or grilled Mediterranean vegetables like aubergines, courgettes and peppers make a brilliant sandwich or pitta filling with hummus or goats' cheese.
> Cooked pulses such as chickpeas, beans and lentils often taste just as good, if not better, cold as hot especially in spicy recipes like dal. They also make a good stuffing for pitta bread (p. 53).
> Baked or stewed fruit can be served hot one day then cold the next.

It's worth taking the opportunity at the weekend to make one or two things ahead that can be used in lunchboxes. A week's supply of hummus for example (see p. 40), one of the fishy spreads on p. 42 and 43 or some homemade soup (see p. 38). A batch of muffins to freeze and use through the week as lunchbox treats. A Sunday night pizza can create leftovers for a Monday lunch.

It also helps to have ingredients in store for those days when inspiration deserts you or you simply haven't had time to get to the shops. Ingredients I find handy to have in the kitchen for hastily whipped up meals of all kinds include:

In the cupboard
Sunflower seeds or some kind of seed mix
Cashew nuts, almonds or pistachio nuts
Dried fruit – such as apricots, dried mango and raisins
Tinned pulses such as chickpeas and red kidney beans
Tinned tuna and sardines
Pasta shapes
Passata
Peanut butter
Marmite
Low sugar muesli

In the fridge
(depending on price and availability)
A lettuce or some kind of salad leaves
Fresh tomatoes
Cucumber
Carrots
Red or yellow peppers } all good for dunking
Celery
Spring onions
Spreadable butter
Organic mayonnaise
Low fat yoghurt or fromage frais
A couple of different kinds of cheese – soft goats' cheese, cheddar and brie usually and a chunk of parmesan for shaving or grating
Eggs
A pack of good quality sliced ham
Lemons
Fresh parsley
Hummus (bought or homemade)
A bowl of home-made fruit compote or fruit salad (see p. 57)

In the freezer
A packet of frozen prawns
Some lean, skinless chicken, breasts or thighs

In the garden or on the window ledge
Chives
Basil

In the fruit bowl
Apples
Bananas
Easy peel citrus fruit in season

Staples I would never be without
Olive oil
Freshly ground black pepper

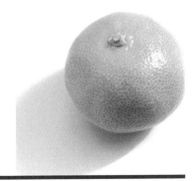

PACKING IT UP

Once your child's lunchbox leaves your hands it may be several hours before he or she gets to open it. During that time it may be kept at a less than ideal temperature so it's important that you try to keep the contents as cool as possible. It goes without saying you shouldn't put anything warm like a recently cooked sausage or bacon in the box and that anything perishable should be kept in the fridge the night before but you can also keep the temperature down by popping a small ice pack in the top or bottom of the box or by freezing the carton of juice you put in overnight. (It should thaw by lunchtime).

Obviously it's also important to keep the box or bag clean which means retrieving it as soon as possible after your child gets home rather than leaving it to fester till the following morning in their bedroom. Any containers or plastic cutlery should also be thoroughly washed in hot soapy water or run through the dishwasher. Plastic bags, foil and other wrapping should be thrown away rather than re-used. You need to get across to everyone involved in preparing lunchboxes (especially teenagers and students) the importance of these basic hygiene rules. (Getting food poisoning . . . missing out on fun at the weekend . . .)

It's worth buying a selection of small plastic containers that will easily fit into a box or bag to keep different foods separate and enable you to vary your child's lunchbox with homemade salads or prepared fruit. They also enable you to pack your own, healthier, less expensive versions of shop-bought products like smoothies, fromage frais and yoghurt.

These containers need to be easy enough for younger children to open at speed but not so loose that the lids leak or come off (particularly important with any container that carries a hot meal like soup). They also need to be of a colour and design that will be acceptable to the junior style police (see Lunchbox psychology). Most supermarkets do a good selection, as do homeware stores such as Woolworths although the cheapest ones may not be the most robust. And Lakeland (www.lakeland.co.uk) has a wide selection available on-line.

A moist-wipe in a sachet and a sheet of kitchen towel are useful additions to clean up messy hands and spills.
> Don't forget to put your child's name somewhere on the lunchbox particularly if he or she has a popular style that looks identical to half a dozen others.

When my youngest daughter was small her favourite meal was what she, more accurately than imaginatively, called 'plate of things'. It was a bright, multi-coloured salad plate with each ingredient cut up and laid out separately – peppers (very popular), cucumber, cherry tomatoes, rolled up ham slices, chunks of cheese, tuna – whatever I had to hand. She painstakingly worked her way through it picking out the ingredients one by one. She loved the surprise of some new element appearing.

I never thought at that stage of translating that approach into a lunchbox but for a small child, about to go to school, it's a good way of getting used to different foods. You could pack it in a plastic egg box or an ice-cube tray, or make a mini version in a quail's egg box. Add a small wholewheat roll and a drink and you've got a balanced meal.

Your 'lunchbox' could contain a selection from any of the following:
> some chunks of cheese – mild cheddar, Cheshire or brie – about 25g in total OR a couple of small chunks of marinated chicken OR a couple of hard-boiled quail's eggs
> cherry tomatoes
> chunks of cucumber, carrot and/or red pepper
> a few grapes or chunks of apple (dipped in lemon juice to stop them discolouring)
> a few unsalted peanuts (provided they're allowed in school) or other nuts and raisins
> a few blueberries, raspberries or small strawberries
> some chocolate or yoghurt-coated raisins or sundried cranberries

Older children are likely to be far too self-conscious to want their lunch presented in this way but may still appreciate a box with several mini containers which separate their food out so that they can see exactly what's in it and enjoy each element individually.

Mini meals
Even the fussiest eater can be beguiled by scaled-down presentation which is a lot easier to achieve than cutting food into shapes. You can make mini sandwiches from slices of bagel (p.39) or mini pinwheel sandwiches (p.38) or make mini kebabs by spearing different foods on wooden toothpicks (cutting off the ends if you fear your child might stab himself or one of his/her classmates). Possibilities include brie and grapes, cheddar and pineapple, Cheshire cheese, cherry tomatoes and cucumber chunks (like a mini Greek salad), cherry tomatoes and mini-mozzarella balls and melon and ham.

Start as you mean to go on. While some small children do develop food fads (my younger daughter had a phase when the only thing she wanted to eat was pasta and sweetcorn) the early years are generally the most receptive in terms of trying new foods so introduce them to as many as possible. You should also avoid giving them a taste for very sweet or salty foods – 4-6 year olds should be consuming a maximum of 3g of salt a day. You can easily exceed that limit in one meal if you buy some of the commercial products which are targeted at children.

Ideas for 'My First Lunchbox' lunches

> 'egg box' with brie, grapes, cherry tomatoes, a small wholemeal roll and water
snack/treat: a small snack pack of nuts and raisins

> tuna and cucumber roll made with ultimate tuna sandwich filling*, little grape and apple jelly*, a yoghurt drink and water
snack/treat: a healthy bar

> mini pinwheel ham and ricotta sandwich*, 2-3 cherry tomatoes, fresh raspberries and a small pot or container of plain fromage frais and water
snack/treat: a snack pack of nuts and raisins

> a small pot of hummus* with carrots, cucumber and mini breadsticks, a mini yoghurt or fromage frais, a few small strawberries and water
snack/treat: a small banana

> 'egg box' with cheddar, apple, cucumber, unsalted peanuts or cashew nuts and sundried cherries or cranberries, a small wholemeal roll and water
snack/treat: a mini blueberry muffin*

> mini 'Greek' kebabs of Cheshire cheese, tomatoes and cucumber, a mini pitta bread, a small yoghurt or fromage frais and a few grapes, a carton of pure orange or apple juice and water
snack/treat: 2 mini date and cream cheese bagels*

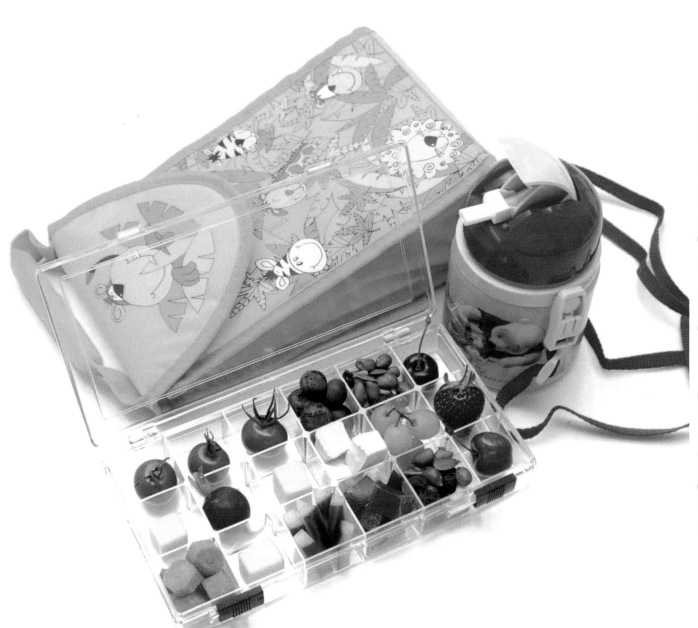

The success of 'dunker' lunchbox products lies in a truth that every parent will have observed: children of all ages love to dip and dunk. There's nothing wrong with that – it's a perfectly healthy way of eating – and a very good way to incorporate veg and fruit into your child's diet.

What you obviously don't want to do is to give them unhealthy things to dunk, salty snacks coated with a cocktail of chemically based flavours. The veg that work best are carrots, celery, cucumber and peppers but you can also lay on lightly steamed beans or asparagus tips, sugar snap peas and baby corn if that's what your child prefers.

You'll also need some carbs in the meal – strips of pitta bread make good dunkers as do breadsticks, especially the ones coated in sesame seeds. You can buy mini breadsticks for smaller children.

In addition to the dips I've suggested you can also make use of the spreads in the book such as the Just-Like-Tuna Pâté on p. 42, the Thai tofu and herb dip on p. 39 or the guacamole on p. 44.

Yoghurt and fromage frais dips are also a way of encouraging kids to eat dairy products and fruit. Strawberries and apple pieces are the obvious choices but you can also dunk pieces of pear, pineapple, plum, melon or any reasonably firm-textured fruit. (It may help your child not to get in a mess if you provide a plastic fork to spear the fruit.)

Although it is easy enough to buy ready-made dips they're likely to be cheaper and healthier if you make your own. A simple mustard and mayo dip for hot sausages can be made by mixing 1 rounded tsp of grain mustard with 1 tbsp mayonnaise. Or you could make a very easy, light cheese and onion dip by mixing a 250g tub of Quark with enough semi-skimmed milk to give it a dipping consistency. Add 2 tbsp very finely chopped onion, ½ tsp garlic paste and a few drops of green pepper sauce to give it a bit of a kick and season with a small pinch of salt. See also tomato and pepper salsa (p. 44) and guacamole (p. 44)

Ideas for 'big dipper' lunches

> hummus* with carrot, cucumber, dukka* and wholemeal pitta bread strips, a yoghurt or fromage frais, a few cherries or grapes and water
snack/treat: 2 mini oatcakes and a small (25g) piece of cheese

> pitta bread with hummus* and grilled vegetables, a blackberry and apple or fruits of the forest yoghurt with some apple pieces for dunking and water
snack/treat: a healthy bar

> Fishy hummus* with pepper and cucumber sticks and strips of wholemeal pitta bread, a small fresh fruit salad and water
snack/treat: A small pack of nuts and raisins

> Just-like-tuna pâté* with carrot, cucumber and radish dippers and breadsticks, an apple and a blueberry mini muffin*
snack/treat: a smoothie

> Thai tofu dip* with cucumber, lightly steamed baby sweetcorn and rice crackers, fruit kebabs and water
snack/treat: a healthy bar

> hot chipolata sausages (from a thermos) with mustard-mayo dip*, some carrot sticks, a few little gem salad leaves, a small roll, an apple and water
snack/treat: fromage frais

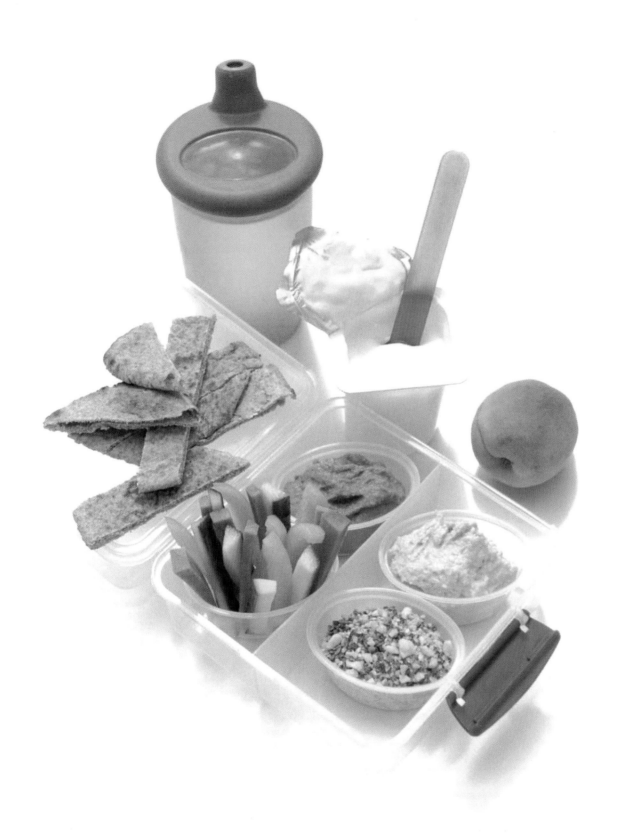

You might say all kids' lunchboxes fall into this category but there are children who find it particularly agonising to stand out from the crowd. The trick is to make the contents of their lunchboxes look like everyone else's while actually being a good deal healthier.

Sandwiches have to be the core of this lunchbox – the big battle being to get your child to abandon white bread. The trick as described on p. 12 is to do it in stages: try white breads with grains and then gradually wean them onto wholemeal. Don't fight on two fronts at once – while you're dealing with the bread issue stick to popular fillings like ham, cheese or chicken – top favourites with kids according to the Food Standards Agency's last lunchbox report. Just try and sneak in some kind of veg.

Crisps are a battle you will have to fight but with any luck the school will do it for you and outlaw them in lunchboxes. Substituting a bag of root vegetable crisps is no help to the self-conscious child. But unsalted tortilla chips might be more acceptable.

Most children are also reasonably happy to munch a whole apple and would rather do that, particularly, when they're older than have you cut it up for them. It's worth trying other fruits from time to time, particularly easy-to-peel citrus like satsumas and clementines in season but there's no harm in sticking to apples if that's what makes your child feel comfortable.

Bars are also a minefield, with an image-conscious child likely to reject anything too conspicuously healthy. The ideal answer is to send them to school with something home-baked that other kids will covet like the home made chocolate and cranberry tiffin on p. 59 or a home-made muffin (p. 60). Otherwise choose something like a Trackers bar – a reasonable compromise.

Appearances are crucial to sensitive kids. You stand a better chance of getting them to drink plain water for example if they take it to school in a sports bottle (let them choose the brand). And let them pick the lunch box or bag they use (see lunchbox psychology p. 11).

If you're desperate for inspiration take a look at the sandwich section of your local supermarket or an upmarket sandwich bar like Prêt. Even apparently luxurious fillings like smoked salmon and prawns are affordable these days: buy the thinly sliced smoked salmon and bags of small North Atlantic frozen prawns as a special treat that should tempt even fussy eaters.

Ideas for 'I don't want to be different' lunchboxes

> tuna and cucumber sandwich made with just-like-tuna paté*, apple, a few Twiglets, carton of orange juice and water
> snack/treat: small packet of raisins

> salmon and cucumber sandwich made with sneaky salmon and pesto spread*, apple, carton of orange juice and water
> snack/treat: a pack of raisins or other dried fruits

> ultimate tuna sandwich*, grapes, carton of apple juice and water
> snack/treat: a couple of cream crackers and a slice of cheddar

> homemade BLT (fry the bacon yourself until it's nice and crisp rather than buying ready-cooked bacon rashers which don't have much taste), grapes, a yoghurt drink and water
> snack/treat: a square of chocolate tiffin*

> cheddar and coleslaw* sandwich (with some extra grated carrot mixed in with the slaw), an apple, orange juice and water
> snack/treat: a homemade flapjack*

> ham and lettuce with Dijonnaise (a mixture of mustard and mayo), a satsuma, yoghurt and water
> snack/treat: a small bag of Twiglets

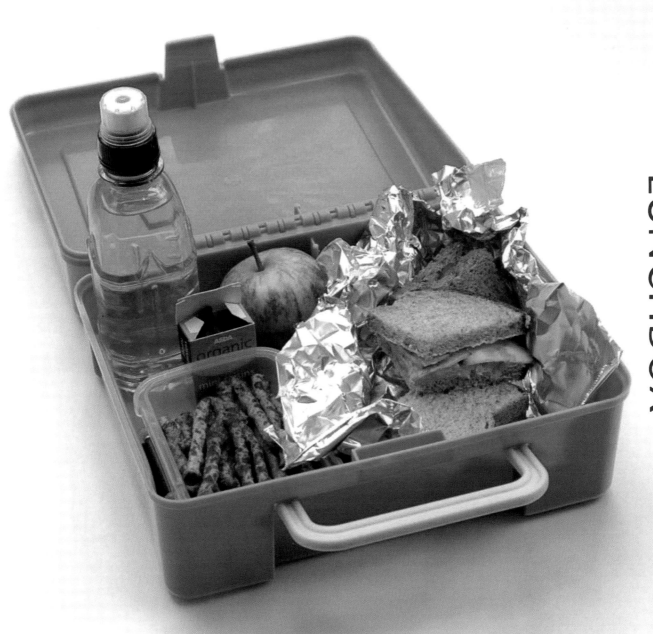

'I DON'T WANT TO BE DIFFERENT'
LUNCHBOX

The idea of an Italian lunchbox may seem a bit off-the-wall but most children love pizza and pasta, and it's a good way to engage a fussy eater. Many of us also eat Italian once or twice a week and a pasta or pizza supper can easily be extended to provide leftovers for the next day's lunch.

In the case of pizza you obviously don't need to make them from scratch although you can control what goes into them and children adore making them. If you buy one ready-made it's better – and cheaper – to get a simple cheese and tomato pizza (with a thin crust) and add toppings of your own. I regularly buy the Dr Oetker's ones (which bizarrely enough come from Germany and are available from many supermarkets including Budgens where I buy them) when I haven't time to make my own and dress them up with additional ingredients.

I have to admit I struggle with wholewheat pasta which I don't find nearly as tasty as authentic Italian pasta but it is worth using it occasionally if only for your kids' sake. It contains more fibre and B vitamins than durum wheat pasta and provides more sustained energy that will keep them going through the afternoon. Tomato-based sauces are much healthier than creamy mayo-based ones which should be kept for an occasional treat.

Both pizza and pasta are high in carbohydrate so make sure the rest of your lunchbox contains plenty of fresh fruit and vegetables. A small green salad and some seasonal fruit such as peaches or melon would be ideal.

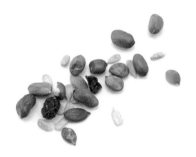

Hot Italian dishes also make a popular addition to a lunchbox. Risottos in particular lend themselves well to being transported in a wide-necked thermos. You can part-cook them the night before and finish them off in the morning or, if you're reheating leftovers, save some of the recipe before it is fully cooked and add extra hot stock to finish.

Chunky minestrone and other Italian style soups make a good hot meal for a cold day. You could even include a hot pasta dish like a bolognese with the sauce mixed in. (Not with spaghetti, obviously, which would be disastrously messy! Use a smaller pasta shape.)

Ideas for Italian-style lunches

> tomato and mozzarella pasta salad*, almost-caesar salad*, melon, red grape juice and water
snack/treat: a mango smoothie*

> a wedge of ham and mushroom pizza*, almost-Caesar salad*, melon and strawberries, plain or sparkling water
snack/treat: a piece of pecorino or other mild cheese and a pear

> tuna and two bean salad*, 2-3 cherry tomatoes, a yoghurt and water
snack/treat: 2 small amaretti (Italian almond biscuits) and cherries

> cheese and mushroom panini*, 2-3 cherry tomatoes, a peach, a small fromage frais and water
snack/treat: a few unsalted nuts or seeds

> ciabatta roll with salami, cheese, tomato and basil (drizzle with a little olive oil rather than using butter or a spread), a small fruit salad and water
snack/treat: fromage frais

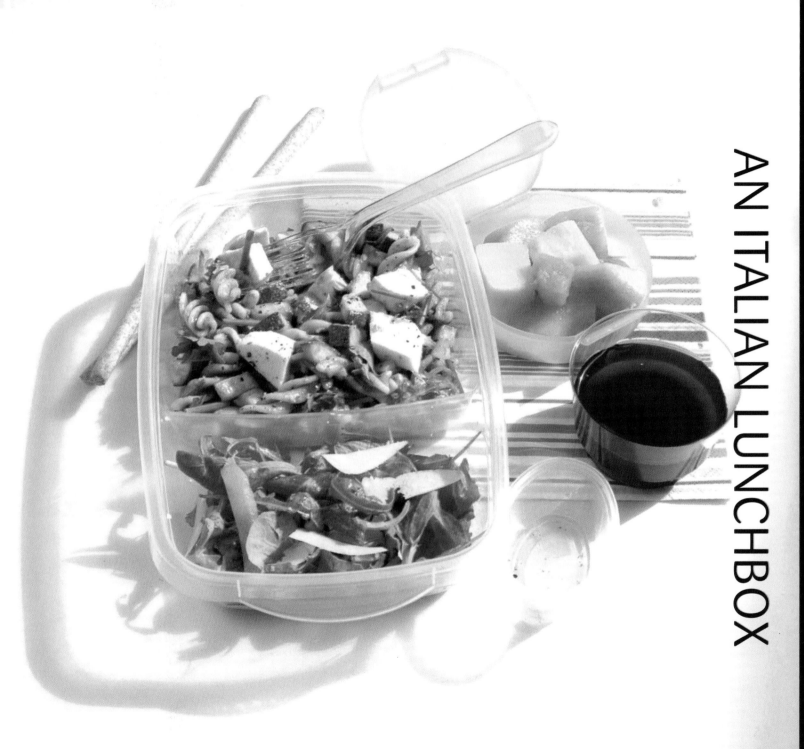

AN ITALIAN LUNCHBOX

Obviously I'm not implying by this that your child should skip breakfast, simply that an all-day breakfast *has* round-the-clock appeal. Just look at the billboards outside any cafe and you'll invariably see one advertised.

What they generally mean by that is the great British fry-up which of course you can't (fortunately) translate into a lunchbox. But the constituent ingredients – eggs, bacon and sausages – can all be turned into healthy meals, so long as you buy good quality ingredients. Sausages with a high meat content, for example.

You can also take a continental spin on the idea, basing your lunchbox on cold meats and cheeses as they do in northern Europe (ham and cheese make a great filling for a croissant) or on an Italian-style frittata* – a great way to use up leftover veg after an evening meal to make a tasty addition to a lunchbox. You can either make a deep (fat) one and cut it into wedges or make it thinner, more like an omelette, and use it to stuff a pitta bread or roll (see p. 52 and 53).

The main challenge with the breakfast idea is squeezing in your child's five-a-day so make sure you include some fruit juice or a smoothie and some fruit. You could include a really delicious fruit pot along the lines of the ones they stock in smart sandwich shops. In fact they're so good the rest of the family is likely to want one to take to work with them too.

Although you can easily buy ready made smoothies it's cheaper to make your own especially if several members of the family are having them. Healthier too. Almost any combination of soft fruit and yoghurt works well but blueberry and banana smoothie and mango smoothie are a couple of my favourites (see p. 56).

Ideas for breakfast-inspired lunchboxes

> Potato, pea and parmesan frittata*, fruit pot*, orange juice and water
> snack/treat: a home-made or shop-bought smoothie

> homemade BLT, satsuma and water
> snack/treat: apple and raisin muesli*

> Egg, sausage and fried tomato sandwich, orange juice and water
> snack/treat: a banana

> cheese and mushroom panini*, 2-3 cherry tomatoes, orange juice and water
> snack/treat: a small pot of plain fromage frais, topped with a few blueberries

> wholewheat pitta stuffed with spicy frittata*, mango smoothie* and water
> snack/treat: an apple

> smoked salmon and Quark (light German curd cheese) bagel, a few strawberries, orange juice and water
> snack/treat: dried apricots, unsalted nuts and seeds

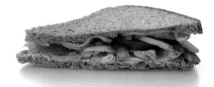

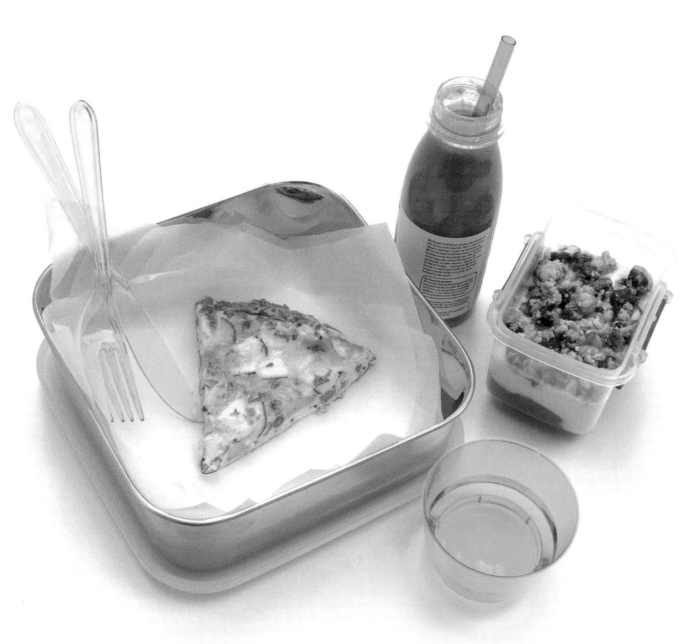

ALL-DAY-BREAKFAST LUNCHBOX

If your child has wheat intolerance you don't need me to tell you that makes the task of providing them with a healthy lunchbox more difficult. Although there are many examples on the market I've yet to meet a wheat-free bread that tastes a patch on a wheat-based version. If the intolerance is simply to conventional wheat you may well find you can make the seeded bread (on p. 59) with spelt. Otherwise it's better to pack non-wheat flatbreads and products like rice cakes with a separate topping that your child can spread on at lunchtime.

It helps to see your child's intolerance as a plus rather than a drawback. That it makes them able to have special food that is tastier and more interesting than the boring sandwich fare endured by their contemporaries. You can do that by making meals that the rest of the family are happy to eat like the Jewelled Rice Salad (p. 48) or an astonishingly Heinz-like tomato soup (p. 38).

Dairy allergies are slightly easier to handle – though can be limiting if they extend to eggs. The best strategy is to try and get your child accustomed to the flavours of cuisines that don't use much, if any, dairy produce – Japanese, Thai and Middle-Eastern food, for example. Again rice and bean salads provide a filling and imaginative meal.

The good news is that many of the bars and savoury snacks that are designed for the wheat and dairy-intolerant are generally a great deal more healthy than conventional ones – well worth incorporating into your child's lunchbox even if he or she doesn't suffer from any allergies. The Village Bakery (see p. 61) does a good selection of healthy wheat-free products. For other suggestions see p. 15.

Although there are now plenty of non-dairy alternatives it's worth seeing if your child can tolerate goats' and sheep's milk products which generally have a more palatable flavour than soy milk or yoghurt. Alternatively you could mix in a spoonful or two of strongly flavoured fruit puree made with dark berry fruits like blackberries and blackcurrants or frozen fruits of the forest.

Ideas for dairy and wheat-free lunches

> Jewelled rice salad*, a satsuma or an orange, fruit-flavoured soy yoghurt, soy milk drink and water
snack/treat: a banana

> tofu dip*, raw vegetables and rice cakes, little apple and grape jelly* and water
snack/treat: mixed seeds

> tomato (and four other vegetables) soup* and rice crackers, a cold gluten-free sausage, an apple, a fruit bar and water
snack/treat: a soy drink and wheat-free cookie

> some cold marinated chicken with black eye bean salsa, soy yoghurt and raspberries and water
snack/treat: oatcakes with hummus* or spreadable feta

> hummus*, dukka* and raw vegetable dippers, a fruit bar, 2 apricots or plums and water
snack/treat: a slice of gluten-free cake

> prawn salad with noodles*, apple and grape jelly*, water
snack/treat: rice cakes with peanut butter

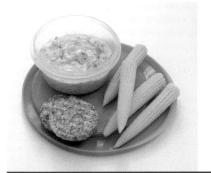

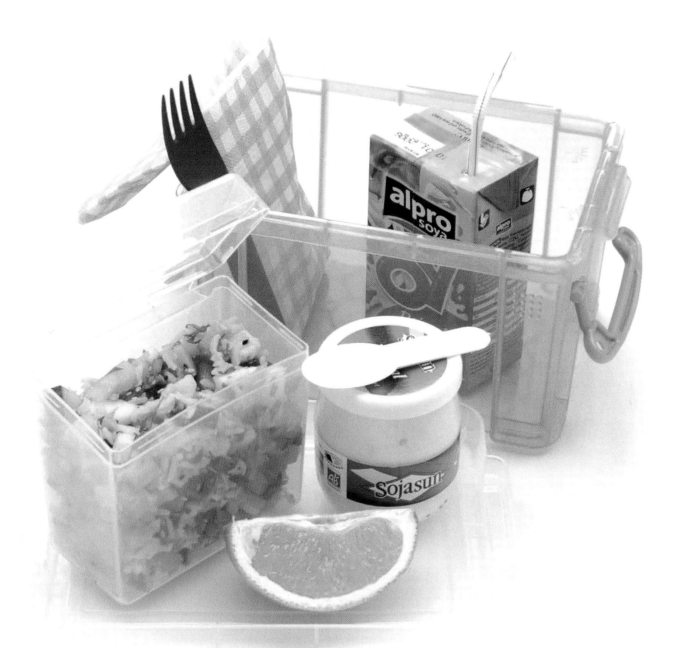

'Green' is shorthand for a whole set of attitudes about food that tend to go together. You may be vegetarian or even vegan. If you do buy animal products such as eggs you insist on them being high welfare and organic. You like to buy locally wherever possible. You support Fairtrade producers. Or you may in the past have done none of these things but suddenly be faced with a child that feels passionately about them.

It's actually incredibly easy now to buy foods that have been ethically sourced. Almost anything you buy is now available in an organic version which means your child doesn't have to be marginalised for their food preferences.

So far as their lunchbox is concerned the crucial thing is to incorporate a good source of protein. For a vegetarian that can come from eggs and dairy products, nuts, seeds, beans, chickpeas and other pulses and soy-based products like tofu. You will give yourself more scope if you can encourage your child to eat salads in their lunchbox as a regular alternative to sandwiches or use cooked beans or pulses as fillings (see pitta pockets with Mexican beans p. 53.)

If they don't eat milk, cheese or yoghurt it's also important to include extra calcium in the form of tofu or soya milk, for example. Chickpeas and sesame seeds are also useful sources. (See also the suggestions in the 'Free From' Lunchbox on p. 28.)

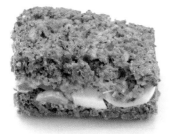

Grow your own

Kids are much more likely to eat herbs and vegetables if they've had a hand in growing them. The most rewarding way to start is with sprouting seeds such as alfalfa which can be grown in a jam jar in 3-4 days. All you have to do is put a tablespoon of seeds in the jar, fill the jar with warm water, cover it with a piece of J cloth or other porous material and secure it with a rubber band. Soak the seeds overnight then drain them. Continue to drain and rinse them twice a day till they're ready.

Ideas for 'green' veggie lunches

> pitta pockets with Mexican beans*, kiwi fruit and pineapple salad, unsalted nuts and raisins and water
  snack/treat: a healthy Fairtrade bar e.g. Geobar

> free-range egg and cress sandwiches made with Easy mix seed bread*, an apple, a yoghurt and water
  snack/treat: a Fairtrade banana

> peanut butter, carrot and cucumber sandwich made with Easy mix seed bread*, an apple, a yoghurt drink and water
  snack/treat: Fairtrade dried apricots and mango strips

> pitta pockets with hummus* and grilled peppers, a fruit pot* made with Fairtrade plums and water
  snack/treat: a couple of squares of dark Fairtrade chocolate and some brazil nuts

> tomato and mozzarella pasta salad*, a small green salad, an apple and water
  snack/treat: a Fairtrade banana flapjack*

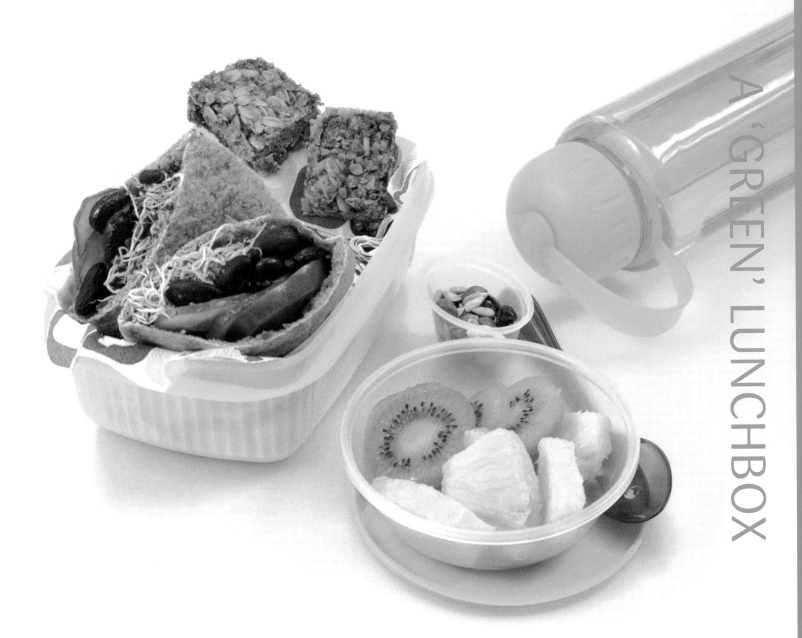

One of the great benefits of taking kids away on foreign holidays is that it gives them a taste for foods they would never eat at home. My normally picky younger son used to tuck happily into wild boar stew when we were away in the Languedoc while his elder brother has retained a lifelong addiction to rillettes and fromage de tete which was known in the family as 'pig's face'.

Family visits to ethnic restaurants can also spark a love of more exotic dishes like crispy duck pancakes, sushi and chicken satay that can be adapted to suit a lunchbox.

You can't, of course, blame kids if they don't respond to these blandishments. Some children are much more resistant to spicy foods than others but it is worth plugging away, particularly if that's the way you like to eat.

The easiest cuisine to start with is Mexican because its flavours are so child-friendly. Most kids love chicken fajitas, an enthusiasm that can be extended to other wraps. Most also like Greek and Middle-Eastern dips such as hummus (see p. 40) and taramasalata and salads made from couscous (see p. 49) which has almost become as popular a household staple as rice. And Indian food lends itself particularly well to reheating if you have a child who is bold enough to take a curry into school. (Cold dal also makes an excellent and nutritious filling for pitta breads.)

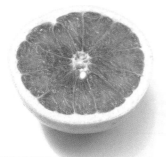

One of the most effective ways to sneak salad into a lunchbox is to make a colourful salsa. Chopping the ingredients up small not only makes them look more appealing it makes them easier for your child to eat without proclaiming that he/she is eating salad. See page 44 for the one I make most often.

Ideas for 'world' lunches

> Mexican: chicken fajita*, crème caramel, satsuma, tropical fruit juice and water
> snack/treat: dried fruit mix

> Greek: hummus*, pitta bread, mini Greek salad, Greek yoghurt and honey, fresh peach or tinned peaches in their own juice and water
> snack/treat: a honey and nut bar

> Indian: pitta bread filled with tandoori chicken and cucumber raita*, fresh mango salad and water
> snack/treat: a small meat or vegetable samosa

> Chinese: hoisin duck wrap*, fresh or canned lychees or a satsuma and water
> snack/treat: a blueberry and banana smoothie*

> South East Asian – prawn noodles*, fresh pineapple salad and water
> snack/treat: a mango smoothie*

> Spanish – frittata made with peppers and chorizo*, a small roll, a small green salad, a satsuma or orange and a yoghurt drink
> snack/treat: a honey and nut bar

> See also the Italian lunchbox on p. 24

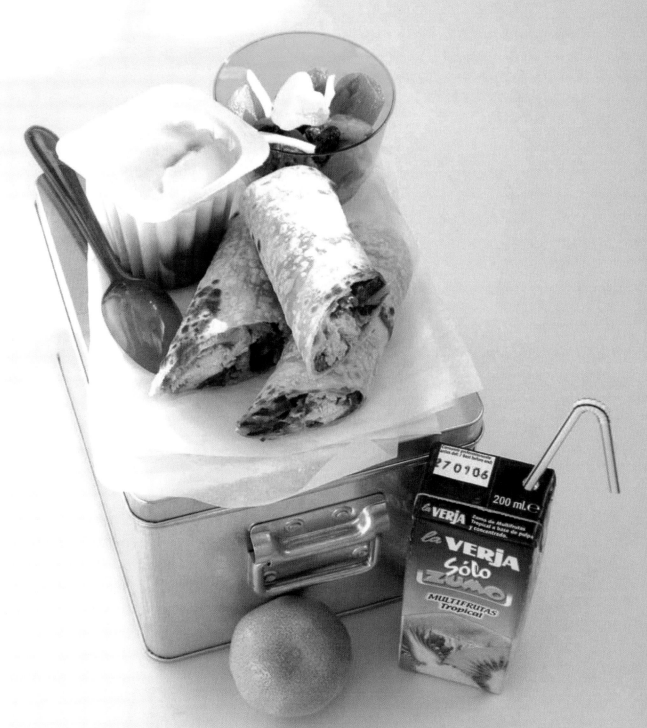

So many teenage girls are now watching their weight. The problem is they tend to do it in quite an unbalanced way – an apple, a couple of crispbreads and a chocolate bar is simply not going to give them the nutrients or energy they need.

Having had two teenage girls myself the answer I believe is to produce light and sophisticated food that they know (because you discuss it with them) is low in fat and sugar – the sort of food that you can buy in Prêt and other smart sandwich shops. Because this is more labour intensive than other foods it makes sense if you get them involved as much as possible in making it and that other members of the family have it too. Not that this is any hardship.

Despite their perception that they need to eat very little teenage girls need substantial amounts of calories, especially between the ages of 15-18 (in fact, more than an adult woman) when they should be consuming 2110 calories a day. They also need higher than average amounts of iron and calcium – iron to compensate for blood lost in menstruation (many teenage girls are anaemic) and calcium to ensure healthy bones and teeth during a period of fast growth.

Meals that are likely to appeal are salads rather than sandwiches, particularly based on what they perceive as healthy foods like lean chicken and prawns, both good sources of protein. Light-textured carbs such as couscous and rice may go down better than sandwiches and combine well with health-giving fresh vegetables and fruit. And there are plenty of low-fat dairy products to provide that calcium boost. You should also try and encourage your child to snack on almonds, seeds and dried apricots, all valuable sources of key minerals.

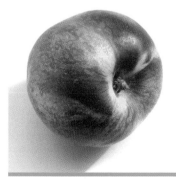

Teenage girls generally need extra iron and calcium. Here's a natural way of making sure they get it.

Iron boosters
Red meat. Mixed bean or chickpea salads, wholemeal bread sandwiches, rolls or pitta breads, sunflower and sesame seeds, almonds, dried apricots and peaches (preferably organic), fresh parsley (easy to sneak into salads), dark green salad veg such as spinach and watercress. Fortified breakfast cereals. Absorption of iron is helped by consuming some vitamin C in the same meal.

Calcium boosters
All kinds of dairy – milk, cheese, yoghurt or fromage frais, preferably in reduced fat versions. Oily fish such as sardines. Dark green salad veg. Tofu, almonds, sesame seeds.

Six ideas for lite lunches that will appeal to teenage girls

> couscous salad with roast butternut squash*, red pepper and feta, little grape and apple jelly*, nectarine and water
> snack/treat: a health bar with nuts and seeds

> sushi salad*, home-made fruit jelly* and water
> snack/treat: a low fat yoghurt or fromage frais

> fruit and nut salad with chicken or prawns* and a small wholemeal roll and water
> snack/treat: a yoghurt and fruit pot*

> Salmon and pesto sandwich with cucumber*, a couple of cherry tomatoes, a home-made or bought strawberry smoothie
> snack/treat: a home-made blueberry muffin*

> prawn noodles*, a fruit and yoghurt pot*
> snack/treat: some unsalted almonds and dried apricots

> Thai tofu and herb dip*, cucumber, carrots and rice crackers and fruit salad
> snack/treat: a couple of squares of dark chocolate and some dried apricots

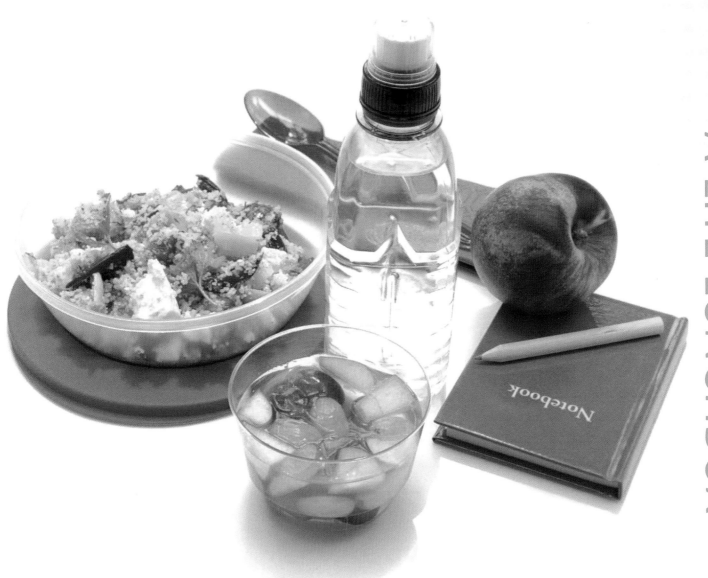

Despite their macho posturing teenage boys can be desperately self-conscious about what they eat. Being seen eating a salad or a piece of fruit is likely to brand you a wuss. You could of course take the 'I don't want to be different' approach on p. 22 but by this age boys need something more substantial especially if they are involved in a lot of energetic sporting activity.

Their capacity to eat can be quite awesome. My stick-thin stepson could easily demolish 15 roast potatoes at a sitting when he was a teenager. Boys aged between 15-18 years need 2755 calories a day plus another 140-odd if they're physically active. They need 55g of protein daily, 10g more than teenage girls. You need to fill them up if they're not to resort to bags of chips at lunchtime.

Unless they're vegetarian (in which case they may have come to terms with eating differently from the pack) large quantities of meat always go down well. If that can be presented in a way that is both acceptable to their peers and which includes some healthy veg (vital if they're not to suffer from hideous adolescent skin problems) so much the better. The recipes for Lean Cajun chicken burgers*, Healthy Chicken Satay* and Slaw* and Chunky Sausage Salad* achieve that aim. Large, well-filled baps, subs or American-style 'hero' sandwiches (hence the title of this section) also go down well (see p. 47 and 55).

It's probably advisable to include cheese regularly as they're less likely than girls to eat yoghurt or fromage frais. And fruit is tricky, barring bananas. Fruit-based drinks like home-made juices and smoothies are likely to be more acceptable, orange and red ones being preferable for obvious reasons to a girlie pink. But if you can't persuade them to eat fruit publicly make sure they get some at home.

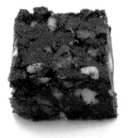

Anything that can be put into a sandwich can be put in a hero sandwich or a sub. They're basically outsize rolls that appeal to outsize appetites. The trick is to layer several different ingredients, meats like chicken, ham and sliced sausage, cheese, egg, salad and pickles. You want to be careful though they don't end up too high in salt or fat so go easy on salted meats like salt beef and salami, pickles and mayo and bump up the layers of salad veg. The Ultimate Tuna sandwich filling* and roast veg and hummus* also make a good sub.

Ideas for 'heroic' lunches that will appeal to teenage boys

> Chunky Sausage and Potato Salad*, a hard-boiled egg, an apple, banana and water
> snack/treat: healthy snack bar

> a large bap filled with a Lean Cajun Chicken Burger* and salad, cheese and crackers and water
> snack/treat: a banana and a healthy snack bar

> 1-2 Healthy Chicken Satay* wraps with Slaw*, an apple, flavoured milk and water
> snack/treat: a chewy banana flapjack*

> a 'hero' sandwich with chicken, ham, tomato and pickled cucumbers, a chicken leg, freshly squeezed orange or pressed apple juice and water
> snack/treat: 2 squares of chocolate, nut and cranberry tiffin*

> 1-2 stuffed pitta pockets with Mexican beans*, tomato and pepper salsa* and unsalted, plain tortilla chips, a wedge of brie and water
> snack/treat: a banana and a yoghurt drink

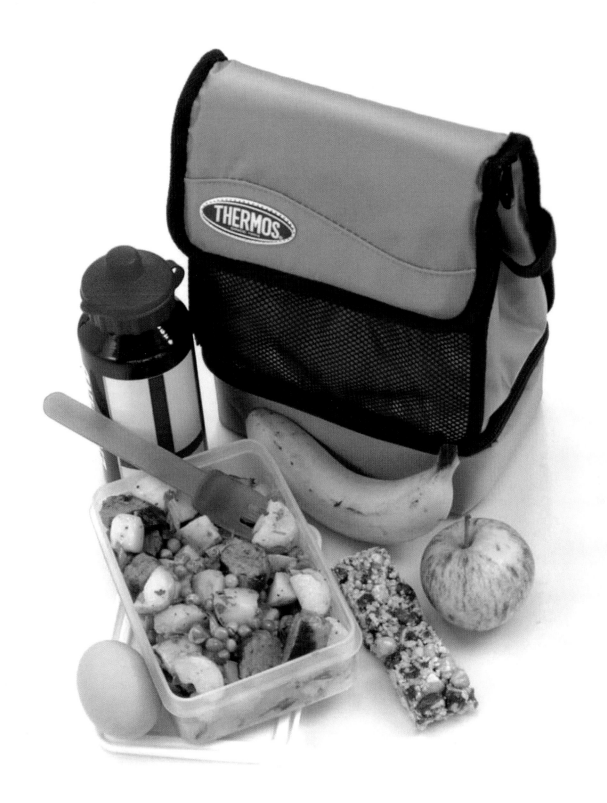

TOMATO (and four other vegetables) SOUP

Uncannily like the Heinz version without any added sugar or salt – or even dairy though it tastes like it. Obviously better made with organic vegetables.

Serves 6

3 tbsp olive oil
1 medium onion (about 125g), peeled and finely chopped
1 medium carrot (about 100g), scrubbed well and finely chopped
1-2 sticks of celery, trimmed and sliced
1 clove of garlic, peeled and crushed
1 medium red pepper, de-seeded and roughly chopped
1 tbsp tomato paste
25g brown rice
850ml vegetable stock made with 1 rounded tbsp vegetable or
    vegan bouillon powder
Freshly ground black pepper

Heat the oil in a large lidded casserole or saucepan. Tip in the chopped onion, carrot and celery, stir well, cover and cook gently for about 10 minutes. Add the crushed garlic and chopped pepper and stir, cover and cook for a further 5-6 minutes. Stir in the tomato paste and let cook for a minute then add the brown rice and stock. Bring to the boil, stir then simmer with the pan half covered for about 25-30 minutes till the vegetables are soft and the rice thoroughly cooked. Leave to cool for 10-15 minutes. Process the soup in batches in a blender or food processor until as smooth as possible*. Return to the pan and reheat, adding a good grind of pepper to taste.

* I say this because some kids object to 'bits' in food and the chunkier it is the less Heinz-like it appears. If you really want to get it super-smooth, sieve the soup setting aside the liquid and process the vegetables first, adding just enough liquid to make a smooth puree then add in the rest of the liquid. Faced with a really fussy eater you can pass the whole thing through a sieve once you've blitzed it.

Per average serving · Energy 110 calories | Protein 1g | Total Fats 7g | Saturated Fats 1g | Sugars 3g | Fibre 2g | Salt 0.5g · **Bonus:** Good source of vitamins including vitamin A for healthy skin and eyesight.

MINI HAM AND RICOTTA PINWHEEL SANDWICHES

Pinwheel sandwiches are attractive and fun for small children to make.

Serves 1

1 slice of wholemeal bread from a medium sliced loaf
1 rounded tsp ricotta or other soft cheese
1 square thin slice of ham
Pepper (optional)

Cut the crusts off the bread and roll the slice lightly with a rolling pin or press it down firmly with the heel of your hand. Spread the bread with the ricotta and lay the ham on top leaving a strip of uncovered cheese at the far end of the bread. Season lightly with pepper if using. Roll up the bread tightly enclosing the ham and press together. Wrap the roll in cling film and refrigerate overnight. Cut it into 6 slices and rewrap.

> You could substitute a thin slice of smoked salmon for the ham or spread the bread lightly with unsalted butter and use one of the fishy spreads on p. 39

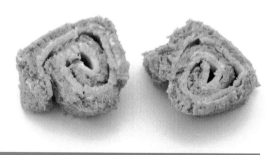

Per average serving · Energy 150 calories | Protein 12g | Total Fats 5g | Saturated Fats 1.5g | Sugars 8g | Fibre 2g | Salt 1.8g · **Bonus:** Good source of protein and B vitamins necessary for active growing bodies.

MINI CREAM CHEESE
AND DATE BAGEL SANDWICHES

Cut a wholemeal or cinnamon bagel into thin slices (you'll have to do this at a slight angle so you get even slices all round). Take two slices and spread one side with cream cheese. Top with a stoned date and sandwich them together. Allow two per child.

THAI TOFU AND HERB DIP

An adaptation of an appealing recipe I found on a Cauldron tofu cookery card. For children with sophisticated palates, admittedly. Very tasty for dairy-intolerant and vegan adults too

Serves 3

125g firm tofu, drained and cut into cubes
½ tsp fresh garlic paste
½ tsp finely grated fresh ginger or ginger paste
Rind of half an unwaxed lime
1 tbsp freshly squeezed lime juice
1 tsp light soy sauce
2 tbsp soya yoghurt
A few drops of green Tabasco or other mild pepper sauce (optional)
2 tbsp finely snipped chives
2 tbsp finely chopped coriander leaves

Put the tofu in a food processor or blender with the garlic paste, grated ginger, lime rind and juice and soy sauce. Process until smooth, then add the soy yoghurt and whiz again. Add a few drops of green Tabasco if using and the herbs and pulse briefly to incorporate them. Good with raw carrot and cucumber strips, lightly cooked baby corn and rice cakes

Per average serving · Energy 170 calories | Protein 5g | Total Fats 2g | Saturated Fats 1g | Sugars 11g | Fibre 2g | Salt 0.4g · **Bonus:** Good source of the trace nutrients manganese and selenium as well as iron.

Per average serving · Energy 50 calories | Protein 6g | Total Fats 3g | Saturated Fats 0.5g | Sugars 1g | Fibre 1g | Salt 0.2g · **Bonus:** Source of minerals such as magnesium and potassium which help to regulate nerve and muscle function.

HOME-MADE HUMMUS

If you're going to make your own hummus you might as well make it from scratch – the taste and consistency is much better and it's much cheaper, if you eat it regularly, than buying it ready-made. It's incredibly easy but does need a bit of forward planning. Start it on Saturday, make it on Sunday and you'll have enough for the week. I like to split the cooked chickpeas up to make two batches with different flavours, each enough for 8 servings.

Basic hummus

250g dried chickpeas
3-4 large cloves of garlic
1 bayleaf
3 tbsp tahini paste, well stirred (about 20g per tbsp)
2 tbsp plain, unsweetened yoghurt
3-4 tbsp freshly squeezed lemon juice
½ tsp ground cumin
½ tsp salt

Put the chickpeas in a bowl, cover them generously with cold water and leave them to soak for at least 12 hours. The next day discard the water and rinse the chickpeas then put them in a saucepan of fresh cold water. Bring them to the boil, skim off any froth, add 3 cloves of garlic and the bayleaf (but no salt) and boil them for about 1½ – 2 hours, topping up the water as necessary, until the skins begin to come away and they are soft enough to squish between your fingers. Turn off the heat and leave them to cool in the pan. Once they are cold, drain the chickpeas, reserving the cooking water and put them in a food processor or blender. Start to process them, adding enough of the cooking liquid to keep the mixture moving until you have a thick paste. Remove half the paste and set aside to make one of the flavours below. To the hummus remaining in the processor or blender add the tahini paste, yoghurt, 3 tbsp of lemon juice, cumin and salt and whiz together until smooth. (If you want to make it more garlicky crush a chopped clove of garlic with the salt.) Check seasoning, adding more lemon juice if you think it needs it. Serve as a dip or a spread.

> If you want to make this dairy-free substitute the chickpea cooking liquor for the yoghurt. You may want to adjust the seasoning.
> You can also add some chopped fresh coriander (about 3 tbsp) to the mix for kids with more adventurous tastes.
> To whip up a quick batch of hummus drain a 400g can of chickpeas and whiz it in a food processor or blender until you have a thick paste. Add 1 clove of crushed garlic, 1½ tbsp tahini paste, 1 tbsp plain yoghurt, 1½ tbsp of lemon juice, 2 tbsp water and ¼ tsp each of cumin and salt and whiz again. Adjust the seasoning, adding a little extra water if it seems too stiff. (Serves 4)

Pink hummus

Whiz two roughly chopped cooked (but not pickled), peeled beetroot in a processor with 3 tbsp of lemon juice. Add half the above amount of cooked chickpea paste, whiz again then add 3 tbsp yoghurt, 2 tbsp tahini paste, a pinch of cumin and ½ tsp salt and process until smooth

Red pepper hummus

Quarter and de-seed 2 large peppers. Lay them cut sides upwards in a baking dish. Slice 2 peeled cloves of garlic and arrange them in the open halves then drizzle over 2 tbsp of olive oil. Roast them at 180 C/350 F/Gas 4 for about an hour until soft and slightly charred. Remove and cool. Discard the garlic and tip the peppers and oil into a food processor. Whiz then add half the amount of cooked chickpea paste above. Whiz again then add 3 tbsp olive oil, 2 tbsp yoghurt, 2 tbsp lemon juice and ¼ tsp sweet pimenton (paprika). Whiz again and check seasoning, adding extra lemon juice to taste.

Basic hummus · **Per average serving** · Energy 110 calories | Protein 1g | Total Fats 7g | Saturated Fats 1g | Sugars 3g | Fibre 2g | Salt 0.5g · **Bonus:** Good source of vitamins including vitamin A for healthy skin and eyesight.

Pink hummus · **Red pepper hummus · Per average serving** · Energy 110 calories | Protein 1g | Total Fats 7g | Saturated Fats 1g | Sugars 3g | Fibre 2g | Salt 0.5g · **Bonus:** Good source of vitamins including vitamin A for healthy skin and eyesight.

FISHY HUMMUS (aka smoked mackerel pâté)

Not really hummus at all but a devious way to get kids to eat fish. Great for grown-ups too.

Serves 8

250g smoked mackerel
250g Quark or sieved cottage cheese
4 tbsp mayonnaise
3-4 tbsp lemon juice
4 tbsp roughly chopped fresh parsley
A few drops of Tabasco or a pinch of cayenne pepper (optional)
Freshly ground black pepper

With a knife and fork pull the mackerel off its skin and flake it roughly. Put the flaked fish in a food processor with the Quark or sieved cottage cheese, mayonnaise, lemon juice and parsley and pulse until the ingredients are just amalgamated. Check the seasoning, adding more lemon juice if you think it needs it and a little black pepper and Tabasco or cayenne pepper, if you want to spice it up a bit. Tip into a bowl and refrigerate until ready to use.

Fishy goings-on

Oily fish, as you know, is fantastically healthy, full of brain-boosting omega 3 oils. The problem is – tuna aside – that most kids won't touch it. Solution: to cunningly disguise it so that it either tastes like tuna or doesn't really taste much like fish at all.

ALMOND DUKKA

This is a fantastic nutty dip that can be eaten in a number of ways. The traditional way is to dip chunks of flatbread such as pitta in olive oil then dip it in the dukka. A more healthy way is to dunk veggies in it like you would hummus (it goes particularly well with carrots and radishes) It's also great as a sprinkle over roast vegetables.

Makes about 250g mix - enough for about 10 servings

125g whole, skinned almonds or nibbed almonds
75g sesame seeds
25g coriander seeds
10-12g cumin seeds
1 level tsp dried oregano
1 level tsp sea salt
½ tsp black peppercorns
Preheat the oven to 180 C/350 F/Gas 4

Lay the almonds, sesame seeds and coriander and cumin seeds on separate baking trays or tins. Roast them in the oven until lightly coloured and fragrant – about 7-8 minutes for the almonds, 5 minutes for the coriander, 4 minutes for the cumin seeds and 3-4 minutes for the sesame seeds. Set them aside to cool. With a pestle and mortar grind together the sea salt with the black peppercorns and oregano. If you feel energetic you can grind the coriander and cumin seeds too (obviously you'll need to do this in batches). Once the almonds are cool chop them roughly if whole then tip them into a food processor. Process them using the on-off (pulse) switch to break them up then add the sesame seeds and coriander and cumin seeds, if you haven't already ground them. Process again till you have a rough textured mixture that looks like coarse breadcrumbs. Add the oregano mix and process briefly again. Store in an airtight tin. (It will keep fresh for 2 weeks.)

> You can use other nuts to make this such as hazelnuts, brazil nuts and peanuts though you may want to adjust the quantity of the other ingredients as they will make the nut flavour stronger.
> You could add some chilli flakes when you grind up the salt and pepper to make it spicier.

Per average serving · Energy 110 calories | Protein 1g | Total Fats 7g | Saturated Fats 1g | Sugars 3g | Fibre 2g | Salt 0.5g · **Bonus:** Good source of vitamins including vitamin A for healthy skin and eyesight.

Per average serving (24g) · Energy 130 calories | Protein 5g | Total Fats 11g | Saturated Fats 0g | Sugars 1g | Fibre 4g | Salt 0.45g · **Bonus:** The seeds are an excellent source of essential fatty acids for healthy skin and nervous system as well as many important minerals such as iron, magnesium and manganese.

JUST-LIKE-TUNA PÂTÉ

This is a crafty way of introducing sardines into your child's lunchbox – by making it taste like tuna

Enough to fill 2 large wholemeal baps, 4 wholemeal rolls or 3 granary or wholemeal sandwiches

-----

1 can of sardines in sunflower or olive oil
75g Quark or low fat curd cheese
Grated rind of half a lemon
1 tbsp chopped chives
Freshly ground black pepper

Drain the sardines, split them lengthways and remove the backbone. (Yes, I know it's healthy but there's nothing more off-putting to kids than coming across crunchy bits of bone) Put the sardines in a blender with the Quark, lemon rind and chives. Whiz, taste again and season with pepper.

> You can of course make this by hand but the extra smooth texture you get from blitzing the mix makes it somehow less sardiney.

(SNEAKY) SALMON AND PESTO SPREAD

Tinned salmon, despite being choc-full of calcium and omega 3 oils is not the most visually appealing of foods but cunningly blitzed into this tasty spread is almost unrecognisable as fish.

Enough to fill 4 wholemeal baps, 6 wholemeal pittas or 8 smaller wholemeal rolls

-----

medium sized (213g) can of salmon
125g drained, tinned chickpeas (½ a 400g can)
2 level tbsp sundried tomato pesto
Juice of half a lemon
2 tbsp finely chopped parsley (optional)
Freshly ground pepper

Drain the salmon and tip it onto a board. Flake the fish roughly, removing any larger pieces of bone. Tip the fish into a food processor or blender along with the chickpeas and whiz until smooth then add the sundried tomato pesto and lemon juice and whiz again. Season to taste with pepper.

Per average serving · Energy 110 calories | Total Fats 8g | Saturated Fats 1.5g | Sugars 0g | Fibre 0g | Salt 0.3g · **Bonus:** Oily fish is an excellent source of essential fatty acids for healthy skin and nervous system.

Per average serving · Energy 60 calories | Protein 6g | Total Fats 2.5g | Saturated Fats 0.5g | Sugars 0g | Fibre 1g | Salt 0.3g · **Bonus:** Oily fish is an excellent source of essential fatty acids for healthy skin and nervous system. This recipe is also a good provider of calcium and phosphorus for healthy bones and teeth.

WHITE BEAN, (MACKEREL), AND CORIANDER SPREAD

Don't mention the mackerel!

Enough to fill 3 large wholemeal baps, 6 wholemeal rolls or 3 granary or wholemeal sandwiches

125g can of mackerel fillets, drained
½ x 400g can of cannellini beans, drained and rinsed
2 tbsp Quark or low-fat yoghurt (about 40g)
2 level tsp coriander paste or coriander in sunflower oil
1 ½-2 tbsp lemon or lime juice
Plenty of freshly ground black pepper

Process as in the previous recipe, whizzing the fish and beans together then adding the Quark, coriander paste and lemon juice and whizzing again. season with black pepper.

ULTIMATE TUNA SANDWICH FILLING

This is my daughter Kate's favourite sandwich filling. (Along with homemade BLTs).

Enough for 1 large wholemeal bap or pitta bread or two smaller rolls or sandwiches.

½ a medium (200g) can of tuna
1 heaped tbsp finely snipped chives
1 tbsp French-style mayonnaise
1 tbsp low fat crème fraîche or plain, unsweeted yoghurt
Freshly ground black pepper
A little grated lemon rind (optional)
1 small stick of celery (about 25g) very finely chopped (optional)

Drain the tuna and tip into a cup or bowl. Mash it up with a fork then mix in the chives, mayo and crème fraîche or yoghurt. Season with freshly ground black pepper and a little finely grated lemon rind if you have some. Stir in the celery if using. Goes well with cucumber, cress or sprouted seeds (see Grow Your Own p. 31)

> It's best to buy tinned tuna canned in spring water rather than oil or brine.

Per average serving · Energy 110 calories | Protein 10g | Total Fats 4g | Saturated Fats 0.5g | Sugars 0g | Fibre 2g | Salt 0.6g · **Bonus:** This recipe is a good provider of vitamin D and phosphorus for healthy bones and teeth.

Per average serving · Energy 120 calories | Protein 12g | Total Fats 7g | Saturated Fats 1.5g | Sugars 1g | Fibre 0g | Salt 0.2g · **Bonus:** Good source of the B vitamins needed for a healthy nervous system and the mineral phosphorus which is needed for strong healthy bones.

TOMATO AND PEPPER SALSA

A Fresh-tasting salsa that may appeal to your child more than a salad.

Serves 4

¼-⅓ of a cucumber
125g cherry tomatoes
½ a large pepper
2 spring onions or a couple of slices of red onion or
    a small handful of chives
1½ tbsp lime or lemon juice
1 tbsp olive oil
Freshly ground black pepper
2 heaped tbsp finely chopped fresh coriander or parsley

Quarter the cucumber, remove the seeds and chop into small pieces. Cut the tomatoes into 4 or 8 pieces. Deseed and finely dice the pepper. Slice the spring onions, snip the chives or finely chop the red onion slices. Mix all the salsa ingredients together and pour over the lemon or lime juice and olive oil. Season lightly with salt and pepper. Add the chopped parsley or coriander just before putting the salsa in the lunch box.
Serve with a fork or use unsalted tortilla chips as scoops.

> You could turn this into a salad by adding a small (300g) can of drained, rinsed black eye beans.

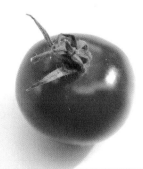

GUACAMOLE

Home-made guacamole is easy to make. Add it to Chicken Fajitas (p.54) or use it as a dip.

Serves 4

1 large ripe avocado
1-2 tbsp lime juice
heaped tbsp very finely chopped onion, spring onion or chives
½ tsp garlic paste
1 tbsp olive oil
few drops of green Tabasco or other mild pepper sauce

Mash the flesh of the avocado with 1 tbsp of the lime juice. Add the finely chopped onion, spring onion or chives, garlic paste, olive oil and a few drops of green Tabasco or other mild pepper sauce and mix in well. Add extra lime juice and a little salt or pepper if you think it needs it.

Per average serving · Energy 80 calories | Protein 1g | Total Fats 7g | Saturated Fats 1g | Sugars 2g | Fibre 1g | Salt 0.4g · **Bonus:** Excellent source of antioxidant vitamins A and C which help support a healthy immune function.

Per average serving · Energy 80 calories | Protein 1g | Total Fats 7g | Saturated Fats 1g | Sugars 2g | Fibre 1g | Salt 0.4g · **Bonus:** Excellent source of antioxidant vitamins A and C which help support a healthy immune function.

QUICK CUCUMBER AND ONION RAITA

Good with spicy chicken.

Serves 4

¼ of a cucumber
2 slices of onion, peeled and very finely chopped
3 heaped tbsp plain, unsweetened low-fat yoghurt
A little salt and a pinch of mild chilli powder

Peel and trim the end off the cucumber, remove the seeds and cut into small dice. Mix with the onion and yoghurt and season with a little salt and a pinch of mild chilli powder.

> If you have time, salt the cucumber lightly and press it between two weighted plates for 15 minutes before incorporating it with the other ingredients. Then rinse and pat the pieces dry. That will stop it making the raita watery. (You won't then need to add extra salt at the end.)

TOMATO AND MOZZARELLA PASTA SALAD

One of the reasons for making pasta salad is that you have leftover pasta. But if you simply use the remains of a cooked pasta dish it can taste unappetisingly heavy and gluey. To make a really fresh, tasty pasta salad you need to measure off the pasta you want for the salad, rinse it under cold water then add some of the sauce you're using for the cooked pasta plus whatever other (healthy) ingredients you have to hand.

Serves 4

100g uncooked weight whole wheat pasta twists
2 tbsp olive oil
1 medium courgette, cut into small cubes
150ml home-made or shop-bought passata
100g mozzarella, cut into small cubes
A small handful each of fresh chives and basil or chopped parsley
Freshly ground black pepper, salt and wine vinegar to taste

Cook the pasta in a large saucepan of boiling salted water, following the instructions on the pack. Drain and rinse with cold water. Meanwhile heat the olive oil and fry the diced courgette for 3-4 minutes until beginning to brown. Remove from the pan with a slotted spoon, cool then add to the pasta along with the passata and cubed mozzarella and mix together. Snip the chives and tear the basil leaves or add the chopped parsley, over the salad and mix again. Season to taste with freshly ground black pepper, a little salt and a few drops of wine vinegar.

> You can vary this all kinds of different ways – substituting a crumbly white cheese like Caerphilly, Wensleydale or feta for the mozzarella, or basing the salad on tuna. You can substitute diced pepper for the courgette or spice it up with a bit of chilli seasoning. If your child has sophisticated tastes olives or capers would be a good addition.

Per average serving · Energy   25 calories | Protein 2g | Total Fats 0g | Saturated Fats 0g | Sugars 3g | Fibre 1g | Salt 0.3g · **Bonus:** Good source of protein, vitamin C, calcium and phosphorus which are vital for strong healthy bones.

Per average serving · Energy 180 calories | Protein 10g | Total Fats 7g | Saturated Fats 3.5g | Sugars 1g | Fibre 3g | Salt 0.7g · **Bonus:** Good source of the vitamins A and C as well as the mineral iron.

ALMOST-CAESAR SALAD

Even a small amount of parmesan cheese makes the world of difference to a green salad; especially one made with bitter (but good for you) leaves. If you can't persuade your child to try them use little gem lettuce leaves instead.

Serves 1

¼ pack of spinach, rocket and watercress salad or other mixed leaf salad
A few fine shavings of parmesan
1 ½ tbsp Italian lemon dressing (packed separately – see below)

Pick through the leaves, nipping off the stalks and dividing up any larger clusters of leaves. (You want your child to be able to eat the salad without great sprigs of greenery falling out of their mouth.) Put in a small container and add a few shavings of fresh parmesan. Put the dressing in another small, sealed container so your child can give it a shake and pour it over when they are ready to eat the salad.

> To make enough Italian lemon dressing for 6 small salads whisk together 2 tablespoons of freshly squeezed lemon juice, ¼ tsp fresh garlic paste, a very small pinch of salt and a few grinds of black pepper with 7 tbsp light olive oil.

TUNA AND TWO BEAN SALAD

A cunning variation on the classic Italian tonno e fagioli, sneaking in some fresh green beans.

Serves 2

75g fine green beans
½ x 400g tin of cannellini beans, drained and rinsed (125g drained weight)
½ x 200g tin of tuna, well drained and roughly flaked
1 medium tomato, quartered, de-seeded and chopped
3 tbsp Italian lemon dressing (see previous recipe)
2 tbsp finely snipped chives
2 tbsp finely chopped parsley (optional)
Freshly ground black pepper (optional)

Trim the ends off the beans if necessary and cook in boiling water for about 4-5 minutes or until just tender. Drain and rinse under cold water then cut the beans into 3 or 4 short pieces and tip into a bowl. Add the drained cannellini beans, tuna and tomato and mix together lightly. Give the dressing a quick whisk or shake and pour over the salad along with the chives and parsley if using. Check seasoning adding a little more lemon juice, oil or pepper if needed.

Per average serving · Energy 130 calories | Protein 2g | Total Fats 13g | Saturated Fats 2g | Sugars 0g | Fibre 0g | Salt 0.2g · **Bonus:** Source of vitamins including vitamin A and C for healthy skin and immune system.

Per average serving · Energy calories 190 | Protein 10g | Total Fats 12g | Saturated Fats 2g | Sugars 2g | Fibre 3g | Salt 0.4g · **Bonus:** Source of fibre as well as the minerals manganese and selenium which are both important for the protective function of antioxidants in the body.

SLAW (OR COLESLAW)

There's something quite macho about coleslaw which makes it a good salad for boys. This is a healthier version which doesn't use so much mayo and also has an intriguingly spicy edge from the coriander. (But don't tell them that.)

Serves 8, more if you use it in sandwiches

½ a medium-sized firm green cabbage (e.g. Savoy) or white cabbage (about 250-300g in weight)
1 large carrot (about 125g), peeled and coarsely grated
1 medium green pepper, quartered, de-seeded and finely sliced
¼ onion, peeled and very finely chopped (about 2 tbsp)
3 rounded tbsp French-style mayonnaise (about 75g)
3 level tbsp low-fat plain yoghurt (about 60g)
2 level tsp coriander in sunflower oil (e.g. Barts)
Freshly ground black pepper

Trim the outer leaves and the hard central core from the cabbage and slice the remaining leaves very finely, using a sharp knife. Put in a large bowl with the grated carrot and sliced pepper. Put the onion in a smaller bowl and mix with the mayo, yoghurt and coriander then pour over the vegetables. Mix together thoroughly and season with the pepper.

> Good with spicy chicken like the Healthy Chicken Satay on p. 56.

CHUNKY SAUSAGE AND POTATO SALAD

This is a real double whammy – a great way of using up leftovers and the kind of meal that appeals to teenage boys who scoff at the idea of salad.

Serves 2-3

3 tbsp olive oil
½ bunch spring onions, trimmed and finely sliced
350g cooked new potatoes, cut into small chunks
110g cooked frozen peas
3 heaped tbsp finely chopped fresh parsley
1 tbsp red or white wine vinegar
4-5 good quality cooked sausages (at least 80% meat), sliced (about 375g)
Freshly ground black pepper

Heat the olive oil gently in a frying pan, add the spring onions and cook for a minute until beginning to soften. Add the diced new potatoes, stir around then stir in the peas and parsley and the vinegar. Leave to cool then add the sliced sausages and toss well together. Season generously with black pepper and toss again.

> **Spicy Spanish-style sausage and potato salad**
You can make a more exotic version of this by frying together a sliced onion and red pepper, adding a clove of crushed garlic, a teaspoon of sweet pimenton (paprika) and a little passata, creamed tomato or ½ x 400g tin of chopped tomatoes. Tip in the potato, peas and parsley as above then once the mixture has cooled add sliced cooked chorizo or other spicy sausages.

Per average serving · Energy 70 calories | Protein 1g | Total Fats 5g | Saturated Fats 0.5g | Sugars 3g | Fibre 2g | Salt 0.2g · **Bonus:** Excellent source of dietary fibre as well as important vitamins such as folic acid, vitamin A, C and K.

Per average serving · Energy 480 calories | Protein 25g | Total Fats 31g | Saturated Fats 8g | Sugars 4g | Fibre 6g | Salt 0.6g · **Bonus:** Source of iron and protein which are both important for growing active bodies.

JEWELLED RICE SALAD

This all-in-one rice salad is a meal in itself but also gives you – or your children – huge scope for creativity. Basically it's stuffed full of fruit, vegetables, nuts and seeds (hence the name). I've given a version below but you can vary it endlessly.

Serves 4-6

110g brown basmati rice
3 tbsp sunflower oil
2-3 tbsp freshly squeezed lemon juice
50g cashew nuts, chopped small
2 tbsp lightly crushed linseed or sesame seeds
25g dried mango strips or halved apricots, cut into small pieces
100g cucumber, de-seeded and diced
A stick of celery, trimmed and thinly sliced
½ red or yellow pepper, cored, de-seeded and diced
1 small apple, quartered cored and diced
2 heaped tbsp finely snipped chives
2 heaped tbsp finely chopped fresh parsley
Salt and freshly ground black pepper

Bring a pan of water to the boil and tip in the rice. Add ¼ tsp salt, stir, bring back to the boil and cook for the time recommended on the pack (about 20-25 minutes). Drain the rice and spread it out into a shallow dish. Leave to cool for 10 minutes then whisk together the oil and 2 tbsp of the lemon juice, pour them over the rice and toss together. Once the rice is cool add all the chopped nuts, seeds, fruit, vegetables and herbs and mix well. Check the seasoning, adding pepper to taste and more lemon juice if you think it needs it.

Here are some other ingredients that you can substitute or add:
Other nuts: walnuts, brazil nuts • Other seeds: sunflower seeds, pumpkin seeds • Other sources of protein: chicken or, if you're not dairy-intolerant, crumbly white sheep's or goats' cheese • Other fresh fruits: oranges, fresh apricots, strawberries • Other dried fruits: apricots, peaches, pears, cherries, cranberries, raisins, sultanas, dates • Other vegetables: finely sliced spring onion (instead of the chives), sweetcorn, cooked peas • Other herbs: dill or mint • Other ingredients: olives

Per average serving • Energy 260 calories | Protein 5g | Total Fats 15g | Saturated Fats 1.5g | Sugars 7g | Fibre 3g | Salt 0.3g • **Bonus:** Source of slow release energy to stabilise blood sugar and control mood also full of immune boosting vitamins.

SUSHI SALAD

My elder daughter Jo adores sushi but rarely has time to prepare it from scratch. This is for her. The logical time to make it is after a meal with rice. Just measure off enough cooked rice for the salad and dress it with rice vinegar while it's still warm.

Serves 3

About 300g freshly cooked basmati rice, white or brown (125g uncooked weight)
2 tbsp Japanese seasoned rice vinegar (e.g. Mitsukan)
⅓ of a cucumber (about 125g), peeled, deseeded and diced
2 spring onions, trimmed and finely sliced
1 stick of celery, trimmed and finely sliced (optional)
200g can of tuna in spring water, drained and flaked
1 level tbsp toasted sesame seeds* (10g)
3-4 slices of pickled ginger (about 7g), finely chopped or a little finely grated fresh ginger (optional)
2 tbsp seaweed flakes or 1 sheet roasted nori seaweed (optional)

Cook the rice following the instructions on the pack. Spread the cooked rice in a shallow dish and pour over the rice vinegar. Mix in well and leave to cool. Add the diced cucumber, spring onions, tuna, sesame seeds and pickled ginger and seaweed flakes if using, and toss together. If you can only find sheets of roasted seaweed, scrunch one up in your hands, scatter the pieces over the salad and stir them in.

> To toast the sesame seeds put them in a dry pan and heat over a moderate heat for 4-5 minutes until they begin to turn pale brown, stirring occasionally. Remove from the heat and allow to cool.

Per average serving • Energy 320 calories | Protein 22g | Total Fats 8g | Saturated Fats 1g | Sugars 3g | Fibre 3g | Salt 1.3g • **Bonus:** Low in saturated fats and a good source of protein. This recipe supplies Vitamin K as well as the mineral phosphorus both important for bone development.

ROAST BUTTERNUT SQUASH, RED PEPPER AND FETA COUSCOUS SALAD

Couscous is now as staple a product in our household as pasta and is even easier to make. Below is the basic method to prepare enough for 2 or as the base for this salad, which is a great way to get kids into butternut squash.

Serves 4

1 small butternut squash (about 750g)
2 large red peppers
1 small to medium onion
3 cloves of garlic, peeled and halved (optional)
3 tbsp olive oil
freshly made up or leftover couscous (see below)
100g feta cheese
4 tbsp finely chopped parsley or fresh coriander
A few turns of a hot pepper spice grind or freshly ground black pepper
A squeeze of lemon

Preheat the oven to 190 C/375 F/Gas 5. Wash the butternut squash, scrape out the seeds and cut each quarter across into 3 chunks. Quarter and deseed the peppers. Peel the onion and cut it into six wedges. Put the vegetables into a large roasting tin, tuck the garlic into the quartered peppers if using then trickle over 3 tbsp of the olive oil. Give the pan a shake to distribute the oil then roast the vegetables for about 45 minutes until soft. Set aside to cool while you make up the couscous following the instructions on the pack. When the vegetables have cooled enough to handle, set aside half the squash for another recipe such as soup and cut the rest into cubes. Mix thoroughly with the couscous. Crumble over the cheese, scatter over the parsley then toss together lightly. Grind over some pepper or hot spice grind and season with a squeeze of lemon (it shouldn't need salt because of the feta).

> To make a vegan version, leave out the cheese and replace it with cashew nuts, chickpeas or pine nuts.
> You could use the rest of the feta to make a Greek salad. Mix it with chopped tomatoes, cucumber, a little spring onion, oregano, oil and lemon juice.
> Another good base for a couscous salad is grated courgette briefly stir fried in a little oil, mixed with prawns, a little chopped mint and a squeeze of lemon. Or cooked salmon, lightly steamed cooked broccoli, and Sunblush tomatoes.

Basic Method

125g couscous
200ml light vegetable stock made with 1 level tsp organic vegetable bouillon powder or an organic vegetable stock cube
1 tbsp olive oil

Pour boiling water on the bouillon powder or stock cube, mix well then pour over the couscous, together with the oil. Leave a few minutes for the stock to absorb then fluff up the couscous with a fork.

Per average serving · Energy 370 calories | Protein 11g | Total Fats 15g | Saturated Fats 4g | Sugars 10g | Fibre 7g | Salt 0.8g · **Bonus:** Superb source of immune boosting vitamins including A and C. Also provides iron which is absorbed more readily in the presence of vitamin C.

FRUIT AND NUT SALAD
WITH CHICKEN OR PRAWNS

This is a slightly ritzed up version of a Waldorf salad, a description I'd avoid using as it probably won't mean a thing to your average teenager. You can also serve it, without the chicken or prawns, as a salsa reducing the amount of mayo and yoghurt to just one tablespoon.

Serves 4

1 medium-sized Cox or Blenheim apple
1-1 ½ tbsp lemon juice
1 seedless mandarin, clementine or a small orange
1-2 sticks of celery (about 50g), trimmed and finely sliced
40g pistachio nuts, roughly chopped
150g cooked lean chicken, cut into strips or 150g cooked, peeled prawns
2 rounded tbsp French-style mayonnaise
2 rounded tbsp plain low-fat yoghurt
A pinch of cayenne pepper or chilli powder
1 heaped tbsp finely snipped chives or dill

Quarter and chop the apple into small cubes. Put in a bowl with 1 tbsp of the lemon juice and toss together. Peel and chop the orange into small pieces and add to the apple along with the celery, pistachio nuts and chicken or prawns. Mix the mayonnaise and yoghurt, season with a little cayenne pepper or chilli powder, pour over the salad and toss together. Sprinkle over the chives or dill and mix again.

PRAWN NOODLES

A simple version of the fantastic spring rolls you find in Vietnamese restaurants – and virtually fat-free. You can make it less spicy if you omit the chilli and fresh ginger.

Serves 2

¼ x 250g pack of fine stir-fry rice noodles
100g cooked fresh or thawed, cooked frozen prawns, roughly chopped
⅓ of a cucumber, deseeded and cut into fine strips
2 spring onions, trimmed and cut into fine strips
2-2 ½ tbsp lime juice
1-2 tsp fish sauce or light soy sauce
1 small mild red or green chilli, very finely chopped (optional)
A little fresh grated ginger (optional)
1 heaped tbsp finely chopped mint leaves
2 heaped tbsp finely chopped coriander leaves

Break the noodles in three and put them in a bowl. Pour over boiling water, leave for three minutes then drain and rinse under cold water. Return them to the bowl and add the prawns, cucumber and spring onions. Pour over the lime juice and 1 tsp of the fish or soy sauce and the chilli and ginger, if using. Tip in the herbs and toss all the ingredients together. Add a little more fish sauce, soy sauce or lime juice if you think it needs it.

> You could use shredded cooked chicken or Quorn in place of the prawns.

Fruit and Nut Salad with Chicken · Per average serving · Energy 210 calories | Protein 10g | Total Fats 15g | Saturated Fats 3g | Sugars 8g | Fibre 3g | Salt 0.2g | **Bonus:** Good source of B vitamins which are needed for energy.
Fruit and Nut Salad with Prawns · Per average serving · Energy 180 calories | Protein 11g | Total Fats 11g | Saturated Fats 1.5g | Sugars 8g | Fibre 3g | Salt 0.4g | **Bonus:** Source of vitamin C and the mineral selenium both of which are needed for a healthy immune system.

Per average serving · Energy 200 calories | Protein 11g | Total Fats 1g | Saturated Fats 0g | Sugars 2g | Fibre 2g | Salt 0.4g · **Bonus:** This is a low fat option for the weight conscious whilst providing the vitamins C and K as well as the trace mineral selenium.

HOME-MADE HAM (AND HOPEFULLY MUSHROOM) PIZZA

You might think with every supermarket selling several dozen types of pizza it makes little sense to make your own but, if you've time, children adore it and it makes for a much healthier meal if you choose your own toppings. Try and sneak in some veggies other than tomato.

(Makes 2 large pizzas, serving 4-6 each)

For the dough

150g strong white flour
100g strong wholemeal flour
½ level tsp fine sea salt
1½ level tsp quick-acting yeast
1 level tbsp sesame seeds (optional)
50ml olive oil
About 175ml hand-hot water
Fine semolina for dusting the baking tin

For the topping

About 500ml home-made* or shop-bought passata
100g sliced mushrooms (if you can get away with it. Otherwise add one of the veggies below)
100g sliced ham
1 level tsp dried oregano or a few grinds of pizza herbs
100g mature cheddar
Olive oil for topping

You will need two large rectangular baking tins sprinkled with fine semolina.
Sift the two flours into a bowl along with the salt, yeast and sesame seeds if using. Mix together then form a hollow in the centre. Pour in the olive oil and half the warm water and stir to incorporate the flour. Gradually add as much of the remaining water as you need to pull the dough together. (It should take most of it – you need a wettish dough.) Turn the dough onto a board and knead for 10 minutes until smooth and elastic adding a little extra flour as you need it to prevent the dough sticking. Put the dough into a lightly oiled bowl, seal with clingfilm and leave in a warm place to double in size for about an hour. Alternatively you can make the dough in a bread machine. Preheat the oven to its maximum setting. Knock the dough down and divide in half. Roll and shape each piece of dough into a large rectangle. Place one of the rectangles on top of a baking tray and spread with half the passata. Top with half the sliced mushrooms and strips of ham, taking the topping right to the edges. Sprinkle or grind over some oregano or pizza herbs then sprinkle over half the grated cheddar. Repeat with the other pizza. Trickle a little olive oil over the top of the two pizzas and bake for 8-10 minutes until the dough has puffed up and the cheese has browned.

To make home-made passata, gently heat 2 tbsp of olive oil in a large frying pan or wok, add 1 clove of crushed garlic, fry for a few seconds then add 1 level tbsp of tomato paste. Tip in 500g chopped, skinned fresh tomatoes and stir well. Cover for 5 minutes to soften the tomatoes then break the tomatoes down with a fork or wooden spoon and simmer uncovered for a further 5 minutes until the mixture is thick and pulpy. Season with pepper and a little salt and cool. (You could also add 2-3 tbsp of finely chopped parsley)

Other pizza toppings:

Courgette, broccoli and mozzarella

1 small to medium trimmed and sliced courgette, about 100g lightly steamed broccoli, 125g mozzarella and 2 tbsp grated parmesan
Pepper and goats' cheese
1 medium to large red pepper cut into strips, 125g goats' cheese and 2 tbsp grated parmesan

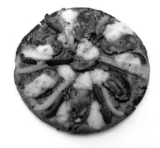

Per average serving · Energy 330 calories | Protein 13g | Total Fats 16g | Saturated Fats 5g | Sugars 2g | Fibre 3g | Salt 1.4g · **Bonus:** Good source of trace minerals including manganese and selenium which are important for immune activity.

CHEESE AND MUSHROOM PANINI

(aka cheese and mushroom toasties, mushroom melt)

A panini is basically a closed pizza sandwich and like pizza tastes almost as good cold as hot.

Serves 3

2 tbsp olive oil
1 large portabella mushroom (about 150g),
   cleaned and thickly sliced
1 sundried tomato or plain ciabatta (about 250g) or 3 ciabatta rolls
6 heaped tsp home-made passata (p.51)
A few basil or rocket leaves (optional)
60g mature cheddar, thinly sliced
Olive oil spray

Preheat a contact (two-sided electric) grill. Heat the oil in a large frying pan or wok and quickly fry the mushroom slices until lightly browned (about 3 minutes). Cut the ciabatta into three chunky pieces then cut each piece in half. Spray both sides of the ciabatta pieces lightly with olive oil. Place them in batches on the contact grill to lightly brown each side. Lay out the pieces, cut side upwards and spread each piece with a teaspoon of passata. Pile up the mushrooms on the bottom half, lay over a few basil or rocket leaves if you have some and top with slices of cheddar. Press the top half of the ciabatta down and put as many of the sandwiches you can fit on the grill at a time, pressing the lid down slowly and firmly. Grill for another 2 minutes or so until the cheese has melted then cool the panini on a wire rack (or eat some and cool some . . .) Wrap in foil.

> You can use almost any kind of pizza topping ingredients for paninis.
> If you don't have a contact grill you could use a frying pan and press down firmly on the panini using a spatula.

POTATO, PEA AND PARMESAN FRITTATA

Although the veg content here is heralded as peas to make it sound more appealing, you can easily sneak in other veggies such as broccoli or try one of the variations below.

Serves 4

2 tbsp olive oil
Half a bunch of spring onions, trimmed and finely sliced
   or a small onion, peeled and finely chopped
   or a trimmed and finely sliced leek
175g cooked new potatoes cut into small cubes
About 55g lightly cooked fresh peas or thawed frozen peas
About 55g lightly steamed broccoli or courgette chopped small
5 large fresh free-range eggs
25g freshly grated parmesan
Freshly ground black pepper

Preheat a grill on medium heat. Heat the oil in a small (20cm) frying pan and fry the chopped onion or leek gently for a minute or two until softened. Add the cubed potatoes, peas and broccoli, stir and heat through without browning for another 3-4 minutes. Beat the eggs, add the parmesan and season with black pepper. Turn the heat up under the vegetables for a minute then pour in the egg mixture. Using a palatte knife or round bladed knife lift the sides of the frittata so the liquid egg falls back underneath. Cook for about 3-4 minutes until the underside of the frittata is nicely browned then pop the pan under the grill for another 4 minutes or so until the remaining liquid egg has puffed up and browned and the top is firm. Slip the frittata onto a plate, cool and refrigerate. Cut into wedges or chunks.

> Instead of parmesan you could add a roughly chopped thick slice of ham or some flaked salmon.
> Alternatives to broccoli would be a small chopped courgette, some peeled and chopped up asparagus stalks, a couple of heaped tablespoons of chopped parsley or, for the more adventurous, a handful of spinach or watercress leaves.
> Make a Spanish-style tortilla by frying together a small onion and pepper (or 100g frozen mixed peppers) with 50g of diced or sliced chorizo, adding cooked potato then following the recipe as above.

Per average serving · Energy 400 calories | Protein 14g | Total Fats 18g | Saturated Fats 6g | Sugars 3g | Fibre 3g | Salt 1.5g · **Bonus:** Provides folic acid which is important for maintaining a healthy circulation.

Per average serving · Energy 210 calories | Protein 14g | Total Fats 13g | Saturated Fats 3.5g | Sugars 2g | Fibre 2g | Salt 0.6g · **Bonus:** Good source of the vitamins A, C and the trace mineral selenium all of which are important for immune function.

SPICY FRITTATA

A recipe for a child with more sophisticated and adventurous tastes.

Serves 2

1 tbsp olive oil
2 spring onions, trimmed and finely sliced
1 small mild red or green chilli
    or a quarter of a pepper, finely chopped
1 small tomato, quartered, de-seeded and chopped
2 tbsp roughly chopped coriander leaves
2 large eggs beaten with 1 tsp of water
Salt and freshly ground black pepper

Heat the oil in a medium sized frying pan until moderately hot. Add the spring onions, chilli and tomato and fry for a few seconds then add the coriander and stir. Season the eggs with a little salt and freshly ground pepper then pour them over the vegetables. Move them around the pan with a spatula, lifting the sides so that any liquid egg runs down to the bottom. Once the egg is set (this shouldn't take more than 2 minutes) slide the frittata out of the pan and onto a plate to cool. Enough to fill 2 whole wheat pittas or baps.

> Columbus eggs laid by hens with a diet fortified with omega-3 oils are a good option for kids who don't eat oily fish.

PITTA POCKETS WITH MEXICAN BEANS

A popular recipe from my vegetarian student cookbook *Beyond Baked Beans Green* which I've toned down a bit for younger tastes.

Enough to fill 4 wholemeal pitta breads

2 tbsp olive or other light cooking oil
Half a bunch (about 3-4) spring onions, trimmed and finely sliced
1 small clove of garlic, peeled and crushed
½ – 1 tsp mild chilli powder
¼ tsp cumin powder (optional)
2 drained, tinned tomatoes or 4 tbsp passata (p.51)
1 x 400g can of red kidney beans, drained and rinsed
2 rounded tbsp chopped fresh coriander or parsley leaves
Salt and lemon juice to taste
Cucumber, fresh tomato and iceberg lettuce or sprouted seeds, to serve

Pour the oil in a medium-sized frying pan and add the spring onions. Stir fry for a minute then add the garlic, chilli powder and cumin if using. Stir and add the tomatoes, breaking them down with a spatula or wooden spoon. Tip in the drained beans, cover the pan and cook for about 5-6 minutes until any liquid has evaporated. Take the pan off the heat and mash the beans roughly with a fork. Stir in the coriander and season with lemon juice and a little salt. Leave to cool. When you're ready to fill the pitta breads pop in a toaster on a low setting, then cut them in half, open them up and leave for 5-10 minutes to cool. Stuff each half with the fried beans and some fresh salad.

Other things you can stuff in a pitta bread:
Falafel, cucumber and yogurt
Greek salad (feta, tomato, cucumber and olives – if your child likes them)
Cold roast or grilled vegetables and hummus
Peanut butter, grated carrot and cucumber

Per average serving · Energy 170 calories | Protein 8g | Total Fats 13g | Saturated Fats 3g | Sugars 3g | Fibre 1g | Salt 0.2g | **Bonus:** Good source of essential vitamins including vitamins A, B and C.

Per average serving · Energy 240 calories | Protein 9g | Total Fats 9g | Saturated Fats 1g | Sugars 4g | Fibre 8g | Salt 1.4g · **Bonus:** Excellent source of dietary fibre which is essential for a healthy digestive system.

CHICKEN FAJITAS

Chicken fajitas are probably my kids' favourite wrap. If you've got any leftover chicken or grilled veg from a barbecue you can make them with that.

1 tbsp oil
1 small onion, peeled and thinly sliced
    or ½ a bunch of spring onions, trimmed and sliced
1 small or ½ large red or yellow pepper,
    de-seeded and cut into strips
4 chapattis or wraps about 20-23 cm diameter
4 tbsp guacamole (p.44) or coriander pesto
200g shredded lean, skinless chicken
A quarter of lemon or lime
A few coriander leaves (optional)

Heat the oil for a couple of minutes in a wok or large saucepan until hot and stir fry the onions and peppers for 3-4 minutes until beginning to brown. Set aside to cool. Briefly warm the chapattis or wraps for a few seconds on each side in a dry frying pan to make them more pliable and leave to cool. Spread each wrap with 1 tbsp of guacamole or coriander pesto, a quarter of the chicken and a quarter of the onion/pepper mixture. Squeeze over a little lemon or lime juice, add a few coriander leaves if using and roll up. Lifting the edge nearest you start rolling away from you, tucking in the two sides of the wrap to make a neat parcel and poking back any ingredients that look like escaping. Cut the wrap diagonally in two with a sharp knife, lightly press the two halves together again, wrap in clingfilm and store in the fridge.

HOISIN DUCK WRAPS

Duck is becoming cheaper and there are often special offers on duck legs. If you roast them, then remove the skin they're perfectly healthy and make a delicious wrap.

Makes 4 wraps

¼-1/3 of a cucumber
2-3 spring onions
3 tbsp hoisin sauce
4 chapattis or wholemeal wraps about 20-23 cm in diameter
200g shredded, cooked duck meat

Quarter the cucumber, cut away the seeds and cut into fine strips. Trim the spring onions, halve or quarter lengthways depending on size and cut across to give you strips about 4-5cm long. Mix the hoisin sauce with 1 tbsp of water. Take a chapatti, spread a quarter of the hoisin sauce over it. Lay a quarter of the duck meat in a thin line down the middle and top with a quarter of the cucumber and spring onion. Carefully roll up the wrap tucking in the ends as you go. Wrap in clingfilm and store overnight. Cut in half the next morning and wrap again.

> You can make another good simple wrap with shredded chicken, finely sliced cucumber, carrot and spring onions and sweet chilli sauce.

Per average serving · Energy 270 calories | Protein 12g | Total Fats 13g | Saturated Fats 2.5g | Sugars 3g | Fibre 3g | Salt 0.4g · **Bonus:** This recipe is low in saturated fats and is also a good source of vitamin B which are needed for energy.

Per average serving · Energy 320 calories | Protein 13g | Total Fats 17g | Saturated Fats 5g | Sugars 6g | Fibre 2g | Salt 1.4g · **Bonus:** Good source of protein and vitamin K which helps heal cuts and grazes.

LEAN CAJUN CHICKEN BURGERS

This recipe unashamedly panders to older kids who are hooked on fast food and is a useful first step in the direction of healthy eating. It makes an ideal mid-week supper with leftovers for the next day. Keep the sausages plain otherwise the overall effect will be too spicy and you can control the flavourings that go into them if you use your own.

Makes 8

3 tbsp olive oil + whatever additional oil is needed
   for frying the burgers
1 medium to large onion (about 150g), peeled and finely chopped
1 large red pepper, deseeded and finely chopped
2 tsp additive-free Cajun seasoning or other spicy seasoning*
375g lean diced chicken breast or chopped,
   skinned boneless chicken thighs
½ x 400g tin chickpeas, drained and rinsed
2-3 skinned traditional pork sausages with a high meat content
   (85% minimum) or 150g of sausage meat
3 tbsp finely chopped parsley (optional)
Flour for forming the burgers

Heat the oil in a large frying pan and cook the chopped onion and pepper on a low heat until soft, turning occasionally (about 5-6 minutes). Stir in the Cajun seasoning and allow to cool. Put the chicken and chickpeas in a food processor and process using the pulse button until roughly chopped. Add the onion and pepper, pulse again. Finally add the sausage meat and chopped parsley and pulse again. Divide the mixture into 8, flour a chopping board and form into burgers about 2 cm thick. The ideal way to cook them is on a non-stick contact grill so they get those appealing stripey lines on each side – about 4 minutes in total. Otherwise cook with as little olive oil as possible in a non-stick pan – about 2-3 minutes each side. Serve hot with baked potato wedges and vegetables or cold in large baps, rolls or halved in pitta bread with salad.

*   You can vary the seasoning in these burgers by using other spice mixes or other vegetables (courgettes would work well). I particularly like the spice blends from Seasoned Pioneers (www.seasonedpioneers.co.uk).

Per average serving · Energy 210 calories | Protein 13g | Total Fats 15g | Saturated Fats 3.5g | Sugars 2g | Fibre 2g | Salt 0.4g · **Bonus:** Good source of the important B vitamins which are needed for energy and for a healthy nervous system.

HEALTHY CHICKEN SATAY

One of my youngest son's favourite meals, this is a lighter than usual version of satay which can be served hot with rice with cold leftovers for the next day. Replace the normal peanut dip with a healthy slaw.

Serves 6

3 tbsp organic crunchy peanut butter
3 level tbsp plain, unsweetened low-fat yoghurt
3 - 4 tbsp cold chicken stock or vegetable stock or water
1 clove of garlic, peeled and crushed or 1 tsp garlic paste
1 tsp grated ginger or 1 tsp ginger paste
1 - 1½ tbsp lime or lemon juice
Hot pepper sauce to taste
4 skinless, boneless chicken breasts (550-600g in total), cut into
   even-sized cubes
Olive oil spray

You will need 6-8 wooden or lightly greased stainless steel skewers. Mix the peanut butter with the yoghurt and enough stock or water to make a thick marinade. Add the crushed garlic and ginger then season to taste with lime juice and hot pepper sauce. Put the meat into a shallow dish, pour over the marinade and mix together thoroughly. Cover the dish with clingfilm and leave in the fridge for an hour or more to marinate. If you're using wooden skewers soak them for 30 minutes in cold water before you use them. Thread the meat on the skewers leaving a little space between each chunk. Preheat your grill to moderate. Lay the skewers in a grill pan lined with a lightly greased sheet of foil. Spray lightly with oil and cook for about 5-6 minutes each side, turning the skewers half way through and spraying the other side of the meat. Cool and refrigerate. You can either pack the satay sticks as they are if you're using wooden skewers or remove the meat from the skewers and pack the chunks separately. Or use them in a wrap with the slaw (see p. 47).

WARNING: should not be given to anyone who is allergic to peanuts.

Per average serving · Energy 220 calories | Protein 19g | Total Fats 15g | Saturated Fats 4g | Sugars 1g | Fibre 1g | Salt 0.3g · **Bonus:** Good source of protein as well as B vitamins which are essential for stabilising mood.

APPLE AND RAISIN MUESLI

There's no need to make this with expensive muesli. A straightforward, unsweetened one with a high proportion of porridge oats works just as well. Makes a good breakfast too.

Serves 1

3 tbsp muesli
About 75ml (5 tbsp) pressed apple juice
    preferably cloudy apple juice
A few raisins
½ crisp apple (e.g. Blenheim or Granny Smith), cored
Plain or soy yoghurt to serve

Spoon the muesli into a small, lidded bowl. Pour over the apple juice, stir in the raisins and leave for 5 minutes. Grate the apple into the bowl and stir then add a little more apple juice if you think it needs it. Top with a dollop of yoghurt.

BLUEBERRY AND BANANA SMOOTHIE

Serves 2

75g blueberries
1 small or ½ larger banana
3 tbsp low-fat yoghurt (sheep's milk yoghurt is good for those who find cows' milk hard to digest)
100g semi-skimmed or soy milk + a little extra if needed
1 tsp clear honey

Put the blueberries in a blender with the banana, yoghurt and honey and whiz until smooth. Add the milk and whiz again. Add more milk if you like to make a thinner consistency.

MANGO SMOOTHIE

Serves 3

1 medium-sized ripe mango, peeled and cut into cubes
250ml low-fat yoghurt
Lime juice to taste
Still mineral water

Put the mango in a blender with 2 tbsp of the yoghurt and whiz until smooth. Add the remaining yoghurt and whiz again. Add a squeeze of lime juice and taste, adding more lime juice if you want it a bit sharper. Dilute to a drinkable consistency with the water.

Per average serving · Energy 180 calories | Protein 4g | Total Fats 1.5g | Saturated Fats 0.5g | Sugars 23g | Fibre 4g | Salt 0.2g · **Bonus:** Good source of iron and the B vitamins which are needed for energy.

Blueberry and banana smoothie · Mango smoothie · **Per average serving** · Energy 260 calories | Protein 2g | Total Fats 15g | Saturated Fats 8g | Sugars 15g | Fibre 2g | Salt Trace · **Bonus:** High in manganese which is important for a number of bodily functions including acting as a protective antioxidant.

FRUIT AND YOGHURT BREAKFAST POT

So much of the fresh fruit that's available is off-puttingly underripe that it makes sense at any time of year to have a bowl of cooked fruit on the go. Ideally that should be based on what's in season – blackberries, apples and plums in the autumn, berry fruits and apricots in the summer but the British fruit season is so short there are going to be times when you need to rely on imported or frozen fruit. (The large bags of frozen berries work well.) Once you've cooked and cooled the fruit you can use it for the basis of this easy recipe.

For each person

2 tbsp plum compote or other cooked fruit (see below)
1 heaped tbsp (about 45g) low-fat fromage frais
    or low-fat Greek yoghurt
1 tbsp (20g) toasted oat cereal (e.g. Mornflake Traditional Crunch)

Spoon the fruit into the bottom of a small lidded plastic tub. Spoon over the fromage frais or yoghurt and top with the toasted oat cereal. Put the lid on. That's it – apart from making sure your child has a spoon to eat it with!

> Cut fresh strawberries, sprinkled with sugar, also make a good basis for a fruit pot.

PLUM COMPOTE

Serves 4-6

2-3 tbsp fruit sugar* or unrefined caster sugar
    (depending how ripe – or unripe – your fruit is)
500g plums, quartered and stoned
1 stick of cinnamon (optional)

Put 2-3 tbsp of the sugar in a saucepan with 100ml of water. Heat over a low heat until the sugar has dissolved then bring to the boil. Cut the quartered plums into two or three pieces and tip them into the syrup along with the cinnamon stick if using. Bring back to the boil then cover the pan with a lid and simmer for 8-10 minutes until the plums are soft. Remove the cinnamon and leave to cool.

* Fruit sugar such as Fruisana has a lower GI (glycaemic index) rating than normal sugar. It's also sweeter so you can use less of it.
> Other good fruits to use are Bramley apples (on their own or with blackberries or plums), rhubarb and apricots.

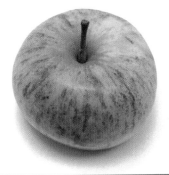

Per average serving · Energy 70 calories | Protein 1g | Total Fats 0g | Saturated Fats 0g | Sugars 15g | Fibre 1g | Salt 0.125g · **Bonus:** Low in fat and a good source of vitamin C for a healthy immune system.

Per average serving · Energy 70 calories | Protein 1g | Total Fats 0g | Saturated Fats 0g | Sugars 15g | Fibre 1g | Salt 0.125g · **Bonus:** Low in fat and a good source of vitamin C for a healthy immune system.

LITTLE GRAPE AND APPLE JELLIES

Jellies are a great way to entice children of all ages to eat fruit. Small children love these miniaturised versions. Weight-conscious teenage girls will appreciate a bigger helping.

Makes 5 jellies

2 sheets of gelatine or ½ a sachet powdered gelatine
300ml clear apple juice
150g green – or black – seedless grapes
1 small to medium Granny Smith or Braeburn apple
Juice of ½ a lemon

Lay the gelatine in a flat dish, cutting the sheets in half if necessary. Sprinkle over 2 tbsp of cold water and leave to soak for 2-3 minutes until the gelatine has softened. Heat the apple juice till just below boiling then take off the heat. Tip in the gelatine and soaking water, stir then leave to cool. When the jelly is completely cold quarter and core the apple and cut it into small, even-sized pieces and toss them in the lemon juice*. Wash and halve the grapes. Fill 5 small containers with the fruit then top up with the jelly. Put in the fridge and leave to set, pressing the fruit down into the jelly half way through the setting time. Cover and store.

* If your child is happy with a slightly sharper jelly you can add some of the lemon juice – otherwise leave it out and save it for another recipe.

Other fruit jelly ideas:
- pomegranate or cranberry juice with fresh or frozen raspberries
- pomegranate and blueberry juice with blueberries
- mango juice with tinned mandarin oranges (in natural juice)
- passionfruit juice with chopped nectarine

FAIRTRADE BANANA FLAPJACKS

One of the best ways you can help Fairtrade producers is by buying Fairtrade dried fruit which you can incorporate into these scrummy flapjacks.

Makes 12 flapjacks

125g unsalted butter, cubed
3 tbsp sunflower or rapeseed oil
125g Fairtrade demerara sugar
2 level tbsp* golden syrup
½ tsp ground cinnamon
100g Fairtrade chewy banana chips (available from Oxfam shops)
200g porridge oats

Preheat the oven to 180 C/350 F/Gas 4.
You will need a small, rectangular baking tin about 26cm x 17cm, lightly greased.
Put the butter, oil, sugar, syrup and cinnamon in a saucepan over a low heat until the sugar has dissolved and the butter melted. Snip the banana slices into small pieces with kitchen scissors. Tip the banana and oats into the melted butter mixture and stir well. Spread the mixture into the tin and press down evenly with the back of a fork. Bake for about 20 minutes until the edges of the mixture are beginning to brown. Remove from the oven, cool for 10 minutes then cut down the length of the flapjack mixture with a sharp knife and make six cuts across to divide the mixture into 12. Leave until completely cold then carefully remove the flapjacks and store in an airtight tin.

> You could replace the banana with 100g chopped dried apple or apricots or replace 25g of the dried fruit with 25g raisins or sultanas.
* Measuring out golden syrup is a bit of an imprecise art. Dip your spoon into hot water first, shake off any excess then take a spoonful, give it a shake and let the syrup fall away. You should end up with about 20g a spoonful.

Per average serving · Energy 70 calories | Protein 1g | Total Fats 0g | Saturated Fats 0g | Sugars 15g | Fibre 1g | Salt 0.125g · **Bonus:** Low in fat and a good source of vitamin C for a healthy immune system.

Per average serving · Energy 260 calories | Protein 2g | Total Fats 15g | Saturated Fats 8g | Sugars 15g | Fibre 2g | Salt - Trace · **Bonus:** High in manganese which is important for a number of bodily functions including acting as a protective antioxidant.

CHOC, NUT AND CRANBERRY TIFFIN

Even a child who hates to be different will welcome a square of tiffin – a wickedly indulgent concoction of melted butter, syrup, chocolate and biscuits. It's also the ideal recipe to entice kids into the kitchen. It doesn't need baking and requires lots of bashing. This is a slightly healthier version using cocoa rather than chocolate, and including dried fruit and nuts but let's face it, it's hardly saintly other than for teenage boys. A one square-at-a-time treat to be metered out during the week. (And that goes for adults too.)

Makes 16 pieces

150g Rich Tea biscuits
75g macadamia nuts
175g unsalted butter, cubed
4 level tbsp golden syrup
3 level tbsp cocoa powder
100g dried cranberries
A lightly greased square, deep cake tin measuring 18cmx 18cm

Put the biscuits into a plastic bag and break up roughly with a rolling pin or the side of a can (you want a mixture of fine and not-so-fine pieces). Roughly chop the macadamia nuts. Put the butter and syrup into a saucepan and melt over a low heat. Sieve the cocoa powder into the mixture, stir and cook for a couple of seconds. Take off the heat, tip in the biscuits, nuts and cranberries and mix well. Tip the mixture into a lightly greased cake tin and press down firmly to even the surface. Cover and chill in the fridge for several hours. Before serving mark the tiffin into 16 pieces. Prise it out of the tin (easier once you've removed the first piece) and return the remainder to the fridge. To transport wrap each piece in foil.

> You could use almonds, hazelnuts or brazil nuts instead of macadamia nuts and raisins, dried cherries, blueberries or apricots instead of cranberries.

Per average serving · Energy 190 calories | Protein 1g | Total Fats 13g | Saturated Fats 6g | Sugars 11g | Fibre 1g | Salt – Trace · **Bonus:** Cranberries are a good source of fibre and vitamin C.

EASY-MIX SEED BREAD

I came across this delicious bread in South Africa and have adapted it from a recipe I was given by the Silwood Cookery School in Cape Town. It's really addictive and ridiculously easy to make as you don't have to knead it. If your kids are into cooking let them do it.

Makes 14 slices and a couple of crusts for toasting

450g organic malthouse or granary flour
50g bran
50g sunflower seeds + extra for topping
15g each poppy and sesame seeds + extra for topping
1 ½ tsp fine sea salt
1 ½ tsp easy-blend yeast
2 tsp barley malt extract (available from health-food stores) or honey
1 tbsp organic sunflower oil + extra for greasing the tin
You will need a large oblong 900g bread tin, preferably non-stick

Tip the flour, bran, seeds and salt into a large bowl and mix together well. (If your flour is cold warm it in the microwave for 30 seconds). Measure out 500ml of hand-hot (tepid) water and stir in the barley malt extract or honey. Sprinkle the yeast over the flour mix and pour over the oil and half the liquid. Start mixing it together, gradually adding as much extra liquid as the flour will absorb. (The consistency should be wetter than a normal loaf – more like that of a fruitcake.) Keep stirring until the dough begins to come away from the sides of the bowl (about 2 minutes). Tip the dough into a well greased bread tin pressing it down evenly. Using a teaspoon gently shake the three seeds in 3 vertical lines down the length of the bread to give you a stripy topping and press down gently. Cover the loaf loosely with clingfilm and leave to rise for about 25-30 minutes until the surface of the loaf is about 1.5cm from the top of the tin. Meanwhile heat the oven to 200 C/400 F/Gas 6. Bake the loaf for about 40 minutes. Using a round bladed knife loosen the sides of the loaf away from the sides of the tin then carefully ease it out and return the loaf to the oven for a final 5 minutes for the base to crisp up. Take the loaf from the oven and leave on a cooling rack until completely cold. Leave it for a couple more hours to firm up before slicing it. (You could freeze some of the slices so they're fresh for sandwiches.)

Per average serving (1 slice) · Energy 150 calories | Protein 6g | Total Fats 4.5g | Saturated Fats 0g | Sugars 1g | Fibre 5g | Salt 0.4g · **Bonus:** Low in saturated fats, high in fibre, iron and the B vitamins, the latter being needed for energy.

MINI BLUEBERRY MUFFINS

Muffins may be the 'treat' in your child's lunchbox but they're not an unhealthy one. They include yoghurt, milk and an egg and are not too sugary. They're also a great way of getting your child to eat fresh fruit.

Makes 12-15

50g butter
50g wholemeal flour
100g plain flour
1 ½ level tsp baking powder
¼ tsp cinnamon (optional)
A pinch of salt
75g unrefined (golden) caster sugar + a little extra for the tops of the muffins
1 heaped tbsp plain yoghurt
100ml semi-skimmed milk
1 large egg, lightly beaten
½ tsp vanilla extract
150g fresh blueberries

Pre-heat the oven to 190 C/375 F/Gas 5.
You will need two well greased mini-muffin tins.
Gently heat the butter in a pan. Set aside and cool slightly. Sieve the two flours into a bowl with the baking powder, cinnamon (if using), salt and sugar and hollow out a dip in the centre. Put the yoghurt in a measuring jug and mix in the milk and the vanilla extract. Pour the cooled butter, beaten egg and yoghurt and milk into the flour and mix in lightly and swiftly with a large metal spoon to get a rough batter (this should only take a few seconds). Tip in the blueberries and gently fold them in. Spoon the batter into the muffin tin and sprinkle each one with a little extra sugar. Bake for 15-20 minutes until well risen and lightly browned. Leave in the tin for 5 minutes then work round each muffin with a flat-bladed knife, ease them out and lay them on a cooling rack. If you're not going to pack them into a lunchbox the same day, freeze them as soon as they're cold.

Other fruit flavours:

> Apple and blackberry (125g blackberries + half an apple, peeled and grated)
> Apricot or plum (125g cut up stoned fruit)
> Chocolate and raspberry (add 2 level tbsp cocoa powder to the dry ingredients and 125g fresh or frozen raspberries to the mixture)

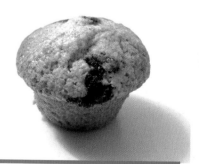

Per average serving · Energy 100 calories | Protein 2g | Total Fats 3.5g | Saturated Fats 2g | Sugars 7g | Fibre 1g | Salt 0.2g · **Bonus:** Blueberries are a superb source of antioxidants which are important for immune function.

USEFUL CONTACTS

More lunchbox inspiration, information and ideas for children's meals:

> **www.food.gov.uk** – the website of the Food Standards Agency has suggestions for a month of different lunchboxes. Also links to a sub-site on the health hazards of salt and how to avoid them – **www.salt.gov.uk** and a helpful site that contains information on how to read food labels – **www.eatwell.gov.uk**

> **www.sustainweb.org** – Campaigning organisation Sustain runs the Grab 5 project aimed at getting primary children to eat more fruit. Directed at teachers but useful for parents too.

> **www.soilassociation.org** – the UK's certification body for organic food. A section of the site is devoted to school meals.

> **www.foodcomm.org.uk** – information about the more dubious marketing practices aimed at children by the large food manufacturers.

> **www.vegsoc.org** – an essential reference for anyone with vegetarian children. Big recipe section.

> **www.nutrition.org.uk** – a good introduction to the basics of healthy eating from the British Nutrition Foundation.

> **www.beyondbakedbeans.com** – my own website – directed at students but with plenty of simple, inexpensive recipes for children who are still at home.

> **www.village-bakery.com** – for a good selection of wheat-free products.

> **www.cwt.org.uk** – the site for the Caroline Walker Trust which works to improve public health through good food and sets nutritional guidelines for school meals and publishes a number of useful booklets.

INDEX

Page numbers for recipes are in bold